KINTSUGI HEROES

Beyond the Deluge:

Flood Resilience Stories from the Hunter Valley

An anthology of stories and experiences from the
2022 Hunter Valley floods.

A Companion Reader to the highly successful Podcast series.

Firsthand accounts of adversity and community resilience.

Copyright © 2024 by Kintsugi Heroes Ltd

All rights reserved. No part of this publication may be reproduced, distributed or transmitted in any form or by any means, including photocopying, recording or other electronic or mechanical methods, without the prior written permission of the publisher, except in the case of brief quotations embodied in critical reviews and certain other non-commercial uses permitted by copyright law.

A catalogue record for this book is available from the National Library of Australia.

This book is dedicated to those people who:

Are experiencing adversity and searching for hope and inspiration.

Want to reframe their thinking to see the hidden value that adversity has brought them.

Want to learn how to better support the people around them who are experiencing life challenges.

ACKNOWLEDGEMENTS

I would like to acknowledge the following people for their contributions to this book.

The Hunter New England and Central Coast Primary Health Network (PHN) for funding the project.

The Kintsugi Heroes who bravely shared their stories to help others:

Annie Cossins, Bernadette Tolson, Carina Moonen, Carly Dawson, Chris Books, Evelyn Hardy, Kirsty McLeod, Leith Moonen, Mick McCardle, Melissa O'Toole, Quinton McLeod, Dr Rob Gordon, Tony Hawkins.

Project partner: Sue George - Manager of the Singleton Neighbourhood Centre.

The book production team:

John Milham - Host, Aveline Clarke - Host, Cecil Wilde - Editor, Patty French - Author, Kate Smith – Graphic Designer, Amira McCue – Proofing

The other members of the Kintsugi Heroes team for their commitment to our mission of:

"Helping people find their own power to heal and to be healed, by exploring their own journey and sharing it with others."

Finally, I would like to thank my wife Helen who has allowed me (albeit sometimes reluctantly!) to dedicate so much of my time, as well as our resources, into pursuing my passion projects and progressing my life purpose.

Ian Westmoreland OAM

Founder – Kintsugi Heroes

TRIGGER WARNING

Some of these stories have themes and discussion around things like trauma, isolation and suicide.

If any of these stories raise concerns with you, please reach out to someone who can support you:

Lifeline
Call: 13 11 14
Text: 0477 13 11 14
Website: lifeline.org.au

Suicide Callback Service
Call: 1300 659 467
Website: suicidecallbackservice.org.au

Beyond Blue
Call: 1300 224 636
Website: beyondblue.org.au

Mensline Australia
Call: 1300 789 978
Website: mensline.org.au

Standby Support After Suicide
Call: 1300 727 247
Website: standbysupport.com.au

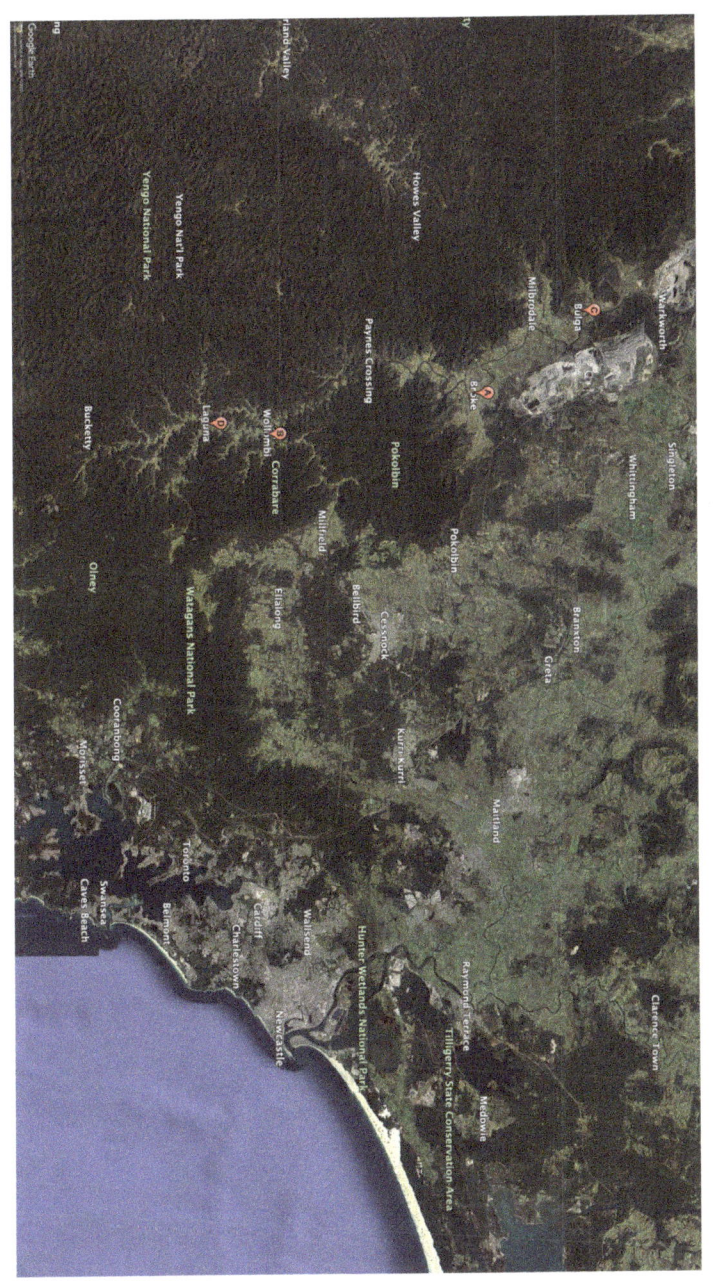

MAP OF REGION

CONTENTS

ABOUT KINTSUGI HEROES 13

ABOUT IAN WESTMORELAND OAM
KINTSUGI HEROES FOUNDER 14

FOREWORD BY JOHN MILHAM 17

    CARLY DAWSON 21

    LEITH MOONEN 35

    CARINA MOONEN 55

    MICK MCCARDLE 65

    EVELYN HARDY 75

    ANNIE COSSINS 95

    CHRIS BOOKS 107

    MELISSA O'TOOLE 121

    KIRSTY & QUINTON MCCLEOD 137

    TONY HAWKINS 155

    BERNADETTE TOLSON 165

    DR ROB GORDON 176

ABOUT KINTSUGI HEROES

Kintsugi is an age-old Japanese art using lacquered gold to repair broken ceramic bowls, bringing them back together as one beautiful piece.

These repaired treasures are considered more valuable and more beautiful than the original. Their gold-joined sections highlight, rather than hide, imperfection.

At Kintsugi Heroes we see this as a powerful metaphor for our own lived experiences.

In overcoming adversity, we can become stronger and more valuable to ourselves, our loved ones and our community.

The stories of the Kintsugi Heroes celebrate the scars we gather over time; the breaks, knocks and wrinkles which create their own unique beauty.

Kintsugi Heroes uses the power of storytelling to provide hope and inspiration to people experiencing life challenges.

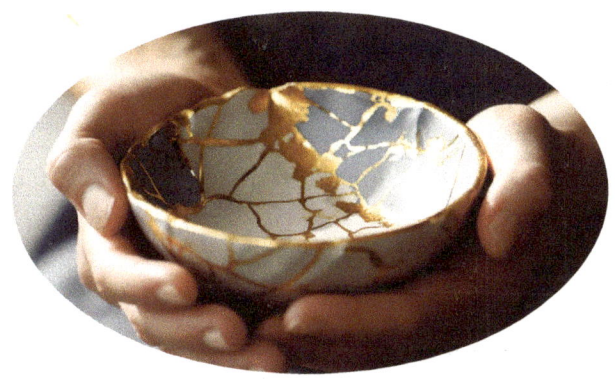

ABOUT IAN WESTMORELAND OAM
KINTSUGI HEROES FOUNDER

Ian spent 42 years working in the Australian and New Zealand telecommunications and energy industries mainly as an IT project manager. In 2013, a profound life changing moment led him to give up paid work and commence a full-time volunteer career.

It was during his work as a volunteer for not-for-profit youth programs such as the Raise Foundation, Kidshope and COACH, Ian noticed a gap for comparable services for mature adults.

However, it wasn't until his own moment of challenge that he realised just how urgently these services were needed, especially for men, a demographic that has historically struggled with vulnerability and asking for support.

In response he developed the Mentoring Men program in June 2018, and it was officially launched as a registered charity by Julian Leeser, Federal Member for Berowra in November 2018. In just three years, Mentoring Men grew to become an Australia-wide, free mentoring service to support men.

With the Mentoring Men organisation now independently up and running, Ian launched another "passion project" called Kintsugi Heroes in 2022.

Complementing his previous volunteer work, Kintsugi Heroes aims to show how those major moments of challenge we face can change the course of our life, making it even more beautiful and fulfilling than ever before.

Kintsugi Heroes is a weekly podcast of inspirational interviews with people who have discovered beauty, despite the incredible adversities they have faced. It's a no-holds-barred approach that does not sugar-coat the difficult road to a life of fulfilment and hope.

Ian's story has been covered on national TV, referred to in both Federal and NSW Parliaments, and included in the best-selling Moments in Time book as well as numerous podcasts, newspapers and radio shows.

Ian and the charity organisations he established have won numerous awards including:

- NSW Volunteer of the Year award 2016 – Raise Foundation;
- NSW Volunteer of the Year award 2020 – Individual and Mentoring Men state finalist;
- AMHF Men's Health award 2020 – NSW Men's Health award.
- 2024 Order of Australia – For services to Men's Health and to Youth

In more recent times Ian has realised how storytelling has played such a big part in his later life, particularly as a father and grandfather.

In one of his favourite photos shown here, Ian is reading Bananas in Pyjamas to a captivated group of four of his grandkids.

Ian has been married to Helen for 41 years and they have four children and 12 grandchildren.

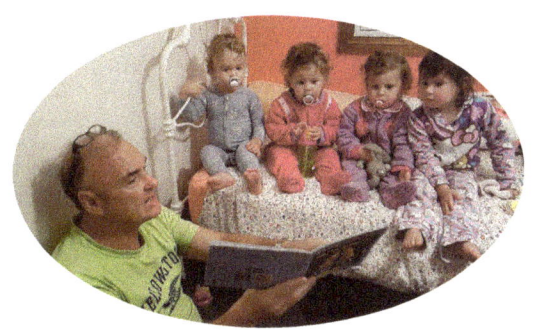

FOREWORD BY JOHN MILHAM

In Australia, it can sometimes feel like there is an unwritten contract we have all agreed to honour, a contract between us, the people who occupy her broad, rich, and beautiful spaces, and our land itself. I feel Australians understand, at some unspoken level, that the riches and beauty of this place are available for our use and enjoyment, but there will be a cost. We have to earn the right to call Australia home.

For tens of thousands of years, Australians have accepted the terms of this contract at the cost of endless hard work, painful setbacks, heart breaking disappointments, loss and suffering. They are asked for resilience and amazing perseverance, and it is all to claim our own little piece of her treasure.

In early July 2022, in a place admired around the world for its rich beauty and natural gifts, the people who live there were asked to endure a heavy cost. Wollombi, Broke, and surrounding local villages were hit by a flood event that was unprecedented in its size and level of destruction. The residents faced a natural disaster on a truly frightening scale, which has become, in some ways, a defining moment for the people and the community itself.

I have been privileged to talk to some of these people—a small number of the many impacted—and hear through them something of their experience, what happened, what it was like, and how it has impacted their lives then and today.

During these discussions, I found myself going back to my childhood memories of being caught up in floods. I lived with my folks in a Northwest NSW town called Wee Waa. It was a cotton town, and my family owned one of the two pubs. It was just a couple of months after arriving that we went through the first of multiple floods over the next seven years.

Our hotel became emergency accommodation, water flowed through our houses and businesses and settled in dark and dirty. Transport became tractor-towed cotton trailers, food and water, and essential services were problematic, and of course, loss was everywhere. Belongings, homes, work, safety, and sadly, sometimes lives. Even now, I cringe at the work it took to clean up and stagger back to normal.

I saw and touched the emotion of my own experience in the tales of the folks in these stories. The trauma they were only just realising existed, the way triggers and fears crept up on them, even today when it rains, or they hear a specific sound. These people stepped up in that moment and moved forward to help themselves and others. They came together to get done what needed to be done.

In doing so, they showed the courage and resilience we acknowledge in this series, something they demonstrated during and every day since the water flowed so destructively through the streets and yards of Broke, Wollombi, and surrounding villages.

We spoke to people in this Kintsugi series who exemplify Australians in a crisis, who were cold, sick, tired, and lost. But they could still step up to care for others, livestock and rescuers. To care for the land and for the community itself.

Through the magic of storytelling, this project aims to help the people who went through these floods (and maybe other floods in other places) to bring some of those fears and triggers to the surface rather than being pushed down to get stuff done.

When we bring that stuff up and let it have its moment, the mind can often let it go, and healing moves forward, because one thing we know is that the contract with our land still holds sway.

I am personally inspired and fascinated by these stories. I love how often people told me, 'Don't talk to me; I did nothing really; it was a bloke down the street who was a real hero!'

Well, I see it differently.

As you may know, Kintsugi is the Japanese art of repairing broken pottery with gold mortar. It is believed that the repaired object with its scars becomes even more beautiful than the original.

So, while events like the hardships of the floods can push us to breaking point, these stories of spirit, courage and restoration can help us cope, heal, and come back stronger as a person and as a community.

I am confident that you, too, will find plenty of inspiration and interest in these tales.

CARLY DAWSON

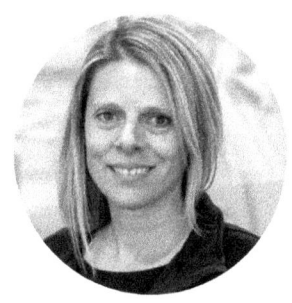

Carly moved to Broke almost a year to the day before the floods. She had been in the area for a while after she and her son had spent a long time travelling and working around Australia in a caravan, but she had no plans to settle in Broke.

Changing circumstances led them to the Hunter, and she subsequently got a job in the Broke area. They had been travelling for about five years at that stage, and it was time to settle down somewhere and try something new. In 2021, she bought an old house in the centre of town.

Carly tells her story with compassion and clarity. The flood did not enter her house but came very close, and she witnessed the devastation suffered by others as she struggled with COVID, so she had to remain in isolation.

'At one stage, I dozed off and woke up much later to a lapping sound. For a minute, I thought I was in a boat because my brain wasn't working properly. I thought, hang on, that doesn't sound good. I went to one of my back rooms to look out the window onto the street, and the water was up around the house. I went out to the front patio, and the water was completely up to the top of the patio stairs.'

Like other locals, she expresses her appreciation of the supportive community in Broke and what that meant to her as a relative newcomer to the area.

We came in on the back end of the 2019 bushfires, about which I heard many stories. That quickly turned into a very rainy year with a few floods before the big one.

For most of my adult life, I hadn't settled anywhere. I moved overseas for a long time and worked in different places in Australia. As a single parent, buying a house was a huge financial and lifestyle change.

But the village was very welcoming. We have a great little village school down the road, and my son was very happy for the week that he was there before we went into lockdown. It was an interesting beginning to our time in the village, that's for sure. But I made some good connections early on.

I love hearing the stories of people who grew up in this area. It seems to have gone through many changes and a lot of growth, especially recently. It's a nice place to spend a while.

I found a job managing an art gallery at a winery up the road in Broke. I was looking for a small farm, but property prices were suddenly booming, and I couldn't afford to do that.

This house came onto the market at the right time. I was lucky to catch it before property prices started to go through the roof. It's a big enough spot for my goats and a couple of other animals, and I can play around with the property.

In the days before the flood, I was busy. I worked at the vineyard and tried to get a lot of work done on this place, which needed a lot of repairs and maintenance, and looked after my son.

The rains had been persistent for a long time.

The previous floods had cut my work off from town, but it was school holidays. I sent my son down to Sydney to spend time with his grandparents so that I could concentrate on work and he could have a little holiday there.

I was alone, and he was supposed to be there for a week or ten days. Then, on the first day, I tested positive for COVID. I was sick and couldn't work, so I was stuck at home for two or three days before the flood.

The floods earlier that year had both cut off the road down to Wollombi; it gets quite deep down there, so when people were saying, 'There's probably going to be another flood.' I thought it was going to cut off Wollombi Road. I didn't imagine that it would be that big.

I was sick, in a fog, sleeping and trying to get well, so I wasn't paying much attention to what was happening around me.

I'd heard it was a big flood in 1949, but from what I've heard since, it was a different type of flood event. It didn't come into the village the same way as this flood. Since then, obviously, the village has grown enormously, and the natural waterways have probably been affected as well. I hadn't heard anyone who thought that the water could enter the village as it did this time.

I was not feeling very well, it was a bad night. The only news I was getting was on Facebook. Whenever I thought about it, I would look up and see what people commented on the notice board.

It was getting dark, and then the electricity went off. It was cold as well because it was winter, so I was sitting by the fire for some light and warmth. I remember there was a message that said the flood water had reached Howe Street. My house backs onto that street, but it was an intersection further down in the village, and I'm higher up.

It didn't seem to be an 'everybody get out' message. I can't remember when we got the message saying to evacuate, but there was nowhere to go by then. The roads were already cut off. You could see on the messages that you couldn't go into Singleton because water cut off the road.

Wollombi Road floods quickly, so you wouldn't have gone there anyway. Then the road out to Cessnock got cut off early on as well. They're all on waterways, so they all got cut off. Then we received a message saying to leave town now. But there's nowhere to go!

I was in a COVID fog and looking at Facebook. I guess I didn't think the water would reach my house. Maybe that was naive of me, but I had no reason to believe the water would get that high.

I kept in touch with my neighbour, who was also on her own, and we had been talking in the days leading up to it.

At one stage, I dozed off and woke up much later to a lapping sound. For a minute, I thought I was in a boat because my brain wasn't working properly. I thought, hang on, that doesn't sound good. I went to one of my back rooms to look out the window onto the street, and the water was up around the house. I went out to the front patio, and the water was completely up to the top of the patio stairs.

That's when I panicked. What did you do at that moment? I called my neighbour, but she was well ahead of me and was outside the evacuation centre at the Community Hall.

She was in her car on the road outside the hall because she had her two dogs with her and couldn't take them inside without an enclosure for them. Although the road was a bit higher, she was worried about how much further the water would rise and whether she would be stuck with nowhere to go.

At that time, no one knew what the water would be doing, and we couldn't get out of town in any direction. When I saw the water up to my patio, I didn't know if it was going to continue rising. That's when I realised, I needed to get out pretty quickly.

I did a lousy job of putting a few things up on a bed, not that I had anything worth saving, and packed a quick bag. I threw in a jacket and some socks that came in handy later.

My car was in the front yard, and the water was already up to the middle of the tyres. I chucked the dog in the car, then opened a gate to get out. I could still see that the road was above the water, but I had to wade through the water, which was very cold and running fast.

I had gumboots on, but the water went straight into them. It was a struggle to get the gate open because there was a whole lot of debris up against it. I got that open and drove out to the road, but I didn't know which way to go because there was water on both sides.

I was sitting up on the road, wondering if I should go towards the store or towards the community hall. All the roads from my place dip down a little bit, so as I sat there, I turned the car around a couple of times.

Then Gary came to the rescue. He worked at the winery where I worked, and he was a hero that evening, rescuing many people. The neighbour I had called at the community hall had gone in and told someone, 'I think Carly needs help.'

Gary knew me, so he put his hand up and said, 'I'll go down and see if she's all right.' He came up and checked me on the road. Meanwhile, another neighbour who also had COVID got in touch and said, 'Look, our house is higher, and it's safe. I've already got COVID, so you can come and stay with us.'

I couldn't go to the community hall. What a complication, being COVID positive! She and her husband have been in the town forever, so they knew which ways they could go where the water wouldn't be too deep.

They came and got me and even rescued my caravan. In the back of my mind, I thought that if the house flooded, I'd at least have somewhere to live.

Her husband said he'd go in and get it as long as I waded through and hooked it up. Good on him! It was challenging to do underwater, but we managed, and I got out to their place. I was there for about a week.

When we returned to my friend Jodie's place, her house was up high, but there was a waterway halfway down her backyard. You could see the water rushing quickly down there. It was intense seeing it like that. It was creeping up the yard closer and closer throughout the night.

I didn't see my house until halfway through the following day when the water had calmed down enough for us to drive through and take a look. That first morning, I was very worried that I was going to go back to a disaster site.

The water didn't get in. It was up to the edge of the door, then it stopped. I don't know how I got away with that. There was an old, enclosed veranda on the back of the house, and a bit lower down, the water did seep into that area and those walls.

But I was already renovating that area. Nothing of any value got damaged and it's all hardwood, so it dried out with fans on it for a few days. There was junk all over the yard, and other things that came with the flood, but the house itself was okay.

My goats were fine, as I had moved them the week before to a friend's property for the winter so that they could be in a paddock with plenty of feed. The goats probably didn't even realise what was happening.

When the water receded, it was shocking to see the damage it had done.

Most people left town the day after the flood. They took them out in buses, and people with bigger 4x4s could go out as well, right past my house. They took their boats out at speed, so all those waves coming up gave us wash damage.

Jody, her family, and I stayed in town. Because of COVID, we couldn't go to an evacuation centre. However, they were set up with enough stuff so we could stay there safely and hygienically.

The water didn't go down for quite a long time; it was still running for that whole first day. It wasn't until the second day that it started to recede. It left piles of junk everywhere. All the fence lines had debris pushed up against them, and there were big piles of sand everywhere.

Some houses were severely damaged. There was a big issue with septic tanks, too, as there is no sewage system, so everyone is on septic, and they're all under water.

Our water got cut off well before the flood came through; when the water breached the road out to Singleton, it also got the mains there. There was no water for a long time unless you had tank water. Even if you had tank water, you needed a generator to run your pump because there was no electricity.

My friends had a caravan with a bathroom that we could use, so we weren't contributing to any hygiene issues. However, the water was not clean, so you didn't want to be going through it, and you needed to be able to clean yourself as well. Luckily, they had a shower in the caravan, so we were able to use that.

We couldn't go to an evacuation centre for supplies, but thank goodness, my friends were very well stocked. Very shortly, as soon as people were able to come back into town, they opened up a crisis centre in the community hall.

We were lucky to have people in the community who provided catering for some time after the floods. Everything in the fridge was damaged, and you didn't always have cooking facilities because the electricity was gone. I suppose you were all right if you had gas.

We were fed well from the beginning and had sausage sizzles from the community groups. Then, they started bringing in supplies and set up almost a shop in the community hall. You could go in and pick up supplies of what you needed, all donated and free of charge. You could also get the basics from there.

Some people were much more affected than others, and almost straight away, those who could help did help. Those who could donate and offer anything were all out there trying to help the situation.

It was brought home what a caring community and village Broke is overall. Mostly, it was all positive. Obviously, people are under stress and in a difficult situation, which doesn't always bring out the best in them, but I found from my experience that it did bring out the best in many people.

I got to know people better and more quickly, going through this crisis together because everything was based at the community hall. Everyone was eating meals together, and you would see people all the time. No one was working, and it was school holidays. Everyone was around, so I formed connections faster than I would have otherwise.

Some people suffered a lot and lost everything. There were people living metres from me who had a far greater impact on their houses and property than I did.

We had these erosion holes, which I'm sure other people have told you about. They're huge holes. We called them sinkholes for a while. We were told that that was wrong and that we shouldn't call them sinkholes because they're erosion holes.

The erosion holes opened randomly. You couldn't tell where they would open. We had one in my direct neighbour's backyard, which opened up two metres from my fence line and swallowed up a carport, an entire car, and a lot of other stuff that he had stored in that area.

I also heard the stories of some of the guys who were out all night with the fire brigade and the SES in the water, putting their lives on the line to help other residents out while their own houses were being destroyed.

It wasn't good seeing the devastation that some people have gone through. Of course, the locals have traditionally joined together in crisis through SES, RFS, and so on.

I couldn't say enough good things about the SES, fireys, and Broke Residents Committee. The council did what they could. Honestly, I don't know how much more they could have done.

Some people were very unhappy with how they handled the issue of stagnant water, and there was a discussion about who was responsible for filling in the erosion holes. I don't know how that was resolved, but it was. I don't know which organisation is responsible for sending out notices to residents. That's something that's been discussed a lot.

I know the Residents Committee has talked about putting together a register so that the community can take advising all the residents into its own hands if something like this were to happen again. The notice that this is quite serious and that you should evacuate came a bit late for most of us.

Help was offered to clean up, but I felt, and many people probably had the same reaction, that I shouldn't ask for help because I didn't get it as bad as the bloke down the road. I'm okay.

I did get the cadets from the Army, who sent through a whole bunch of people. We have the training grounds down the road, so they sent a group of guys to wander the street to help anyone who needed it. They helped me clear stuff out of my yard that I couldn't do on my own.

There were also the mines. They rostered people for the Broke clean-up duty. That was their shift for the day, and they would wander around helping.

People could go to the community hall and put their names on a list and a job they needed to be done. The guys organising that area were sending out people to do jobs that needed to be done—ripping up carpet, clearing out furniture, helping clean up debris or demolishing things. That was a lot of work, and they organised the septic clean-up. They had a roster, and they'd give you a call and say, 'Hey, we're sending someone over now.'

As much as we got good support and a good community that came together, it was still a traumatic experience. For quite some time afterwards, if it ever rained heavily, you panicked a bit, wondering—what if it ever happened again?

I was trying to help a family I knew before this happened. Their situation was the most challenging part of the whole thing. In some ways, they slipped through the cracks as part of the community but didn't have all the same help available.

How did that happen? Some people were outliers or didn't fit the normal thing regarding getting real support when you lose everything. There was support out there for homeowners with insurance and support for homeowners who didn't have insurance. There were emergency payments. You could even get some wages paid out to you. There were emergency and crisis payments and help out there. But you could easily be left out if you didn't fit the criteria.

The family I'm referring to had lived in Broke for a few years. They were renting a place that got completely flooded to within 20 centimetres of the ceiling inside. They lost everything, and unfortunately, the father was sick at the time.

They couldn't be prepared enough to put everything together and get out. They evacuated to a house on higher ground, up from where their house was, and could see their belongings floating down the river in front of them, but they couldn't do a thing about it.

They came from New Zealand originally, with three children. But they didn't own a house, and they couldn't go back to their rental, which wouldn't be rebuilt afterwards. Only one of them had been working in Australia long enough to be eligible for the emergency payment.

The only option given to them was crisis accommodation. It was ten days of accommodation in Singleton. Two rooms at a roadside motel with no cooking facilities, and three kids at school, and they had lost everything.

They had to apply for ten more days each time it ran out, and it wasn't necessarily going to be in the same place or have the same rooms. Every ten days, they would potentially have to move or not, but they didn't know.

I helped them as much as I could by calling around and seeing their options. There was little help the government systems could offer them. Someone suggested a caravan, and I said, 'Well, they can stay at my place.' Then, a lovely local family lent them their caravan to live in. I set it up on my block, and they moved in there.

The Residents Committee did a lot of fundraising for the people who lost everything, and I know they helped this family rebuild their lives and replace some of the things that they'd lost, but it was left to the community to look after people like that.

There are probably other similar stories in Broke. This is the one that I know about.

Walking around and seeing people's lives in a pile outside the house was pretty wild.

The worst thing about it is when people come in to do crisis tourism. Being in a tourism area, we couldn't stop them from coming through. They closed the streets into the village to non-residents, but there were definitely people who came around to sticky beak.

The piles were a topic for a while because people were coming in and going through them to try and salvage things. Some people looked at it almost as a council clean-up; if it's out there, you can reuse and recycle things. That's all good, but it was not the time or place to do that.

It would be contaminated if it was in the floodwater, so you wouldn't want it anyway. But if it's your personal items that you're putting out there only because of this horrible tragedy, then having people rifle through them is very uncomfortable. It's not the way it should be.

Recovery took a long time, which also applies to the piles of rubbish; they took a long time to disappear. It is not easy to start thinking about what comes next when you're looking at the remnants of what was before every day.

That goes for the piles and erosion holes. A car stuck out of a hole in my yard for weeks afterwards. The stagnant water became a real issue because people wanted to pump it out of their properties, but they would pump it out, and it would end up on someone else's property. The cleaning-up process was very long and drawn out.

It's been a different journey for everyone. Some people had far more traumatic experiences than others. I was having a hard time thinking about going back to work afterwards and having to talk to tourists quite soon after the floods. I knew there would be many well-intentioned questions—'How did you go? Are you okay? Oh, what happened?'

You understand why people want to ask these questions, but it would have meant me talking about the destruction of my neighbours, houses and lives. I didn't end up going back to work there. I found another job.

I've wanted to have conversations with people who also experienced it, and there was a lot of that. Maybe not for everyone, but my experience with the people I encountered was wanting to share stories and hear other people's stories. I think it helps.

Initially, there was a divide between the people who were out of the village and the people in the village and between people who thought that help was focused on one area and not another. But, after the initial chaos cleared up, there were community meetings with much discussion afterwards.

Broke is changing. From what I've heard from people who have lived here much longer than I have, it's gone through much change. It's growing.

There's a bit of movement in properties and population.

I hope that, because I think it's a question of when it happens again, it will be managed differently before the flood happens rather than afterwards. There was a lot of good management after the flood. I believe that we probably fared better than other communities that have gone through big floods, especially during that year when the floods up north happened. I think we're lucky in that sense that we had more services directly surrounding our community that got in straight away and helped us out. I hope that with our early warning system being set up, better prevention will be possible in the future.

I think everyone knows it will happen again.

When I got a new hot water system installed, I said, 'Oh, you need to make sure that it's put in above a certain level because it will flood, and I don't want that to get damaged.' It's always in the back of your head that whatever we do from here on, we want to minimise any future damage.

In the end, if the stuff in the house gets damaged, it would be awful, but it would be okay again. What matters is being looked after in the first few days afterwards, and then being able to help look after other people as well.

CARLY DAWSON

BEYOND THE DELUGE

LEITH MOONEN

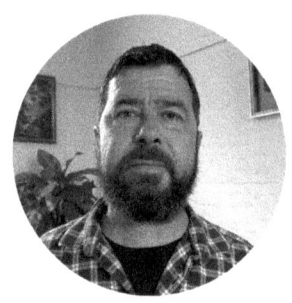

Leith tells his story about the 6th of July, when he and his wife, Carina, were caught up in the floods in a dramatic fashion.

Their village, Warkworth, was out of the way and not part of the hub of activity, but they were heavily impacted on the day of the flood. They lost many valuable possessions and personal treasures.

'Unfortunately, the short-term goal of this situation is to raise awareness of many of these issues and find out why people like us were forgotten.'

'We had no communication to know what other people were doing apart from people stopping by. We saw no emergency services. We had nothing. We had no information besides this water is in our house now. The only assistance we received was from some community people and a couple of stubborn mates who drove out to help out. The area was shut, locked down with floods happening all around.'

'If people want to help, the help has to be appropriate. Sometimes, it's not. Some people can hinder, and some people can help.'

'Certain things keep taking you back every time. Some of them are the sounds that trigger you. Even leading up to this discussion, I've started having dreams again. The other night, I was running around trying to save everything, and I couldn't because we were in a washing machine— even the car was in there. It's sights and sounds that trigger these things'.

My wife Carina and I and our son Sean lived at Warkworth in the old rural schoolhouse for around 20 years. It was built around 1859 and closed around 1997.

I've spent a lot of time in the riverbed there as you do when you've got a young fella growing up. We spent a lot of time down there fishing, exploring, catching fish. As he got older, he'd do it himself down there.

We know the river quite well and have watched it flood numerous times. Prior to flooding, it tends to sit at a higher level for quite some time. I thought it would go down this time, as it has happened many times since we've lived there. A fairly low-scale flood usually passes quickly.

I'm told that the Lombard Brook is one of the fastest flowing sand bed riverbeds in the Southern Hemisphere. I do not know if that's true, but I heard that from a mate's dad, and they are long-term Broke residents.

I've seen it flow very fast and very slowly in floods. But it will usually sit around a metre higher than usual. That's what it has done in every flood in history that I can find in my records dating back to 1908. The trend is a metre higher for around six months before these flood events.

If it's not sitting at that level, the water table is nice and low and tends to soak in quickly. There was a lot of rain leading up to this after a drought.

We had severe floods before July, but the difference was in the rain events and storms leading up to them. Many of the gullies in the mountains had opened up, so there was no restriction on the water flow. It came out much faster than expected and was timed perfectly for the flood, but not for us.

We expected a flood, but this one was unexpected in its severity and speed.

Wollombi and Broke river systems are big catchments for the whole valley. The water starts off at the back of the Central Coast, up on Mangrove Mountain.

That river is very healthy. Many people will look at it and say, 'Oh, there's no water flowing,' but that's only what they can see on either side of the bridge next to our house on the Golden Highway. If you look down, you can't see much water, just a little stream on the side. That's where the historical crossings were, and they've put a lot of gravel into the riverbed. There are some good holes 50 meters on either side of there. The riverbed is predominantly sand, but there's a lot of rock. When it floods like this, unlike sand, it doesn't change.

I've seen photos downstream from our house in the 1950s, and it's very wide and open. That was after two periods of flooding, the 1949 and 1955 floods. They opened up the channel very wide, which is unhealthy for a riverbed and leads to much erosion.

A lot of the bank was lost, but now it's starting to recover. There's vegetation on the banks, and it's held together really well. It looks no different, with a few logs sticking up in the trees, providing evidence of a flood.

The best thing about living here is that I can go for a walk along the creek, sit down and take in the birds and all the nature.

A wise man once walked past me while I was fishing in very poor weather. He said to me, 'It's not a good day for fishing.' I was not having a good day, but I looked at him and said, 'Look, mate, sometimes fishing is not about catching fish.'

He just smiled, nodded and wandered off.

Prior to the flood, we were quite comfortable. We were starting to downsize a lot of stuff to de-clutter from living in one place for 20-odd years.

We're not spring chickens anymore. We had plans for the future and were quite comfortable and complacent. My wife had a workplace injury, so she was currently on Workers Comp, which was the only negative at the time.

On Christmas day, 2021, everything was going along quite well, but then the police arrived at the gate to tell me my father had passed away.

After that, nothing in life went to plan. It is now two and a half years after the flood, and still nothing's going to plan.

Everything I went to do, something would go wrong. I go to fix something in the shed, then realise I no longer have the tools to do this job. I also lost my little dog, who was about to turn 20, on Valentine's Day 2022.

When we lost her, we thought, bugger it, let's cheer up by celebrating Christmas in July. The whole family was keen to have a Christmas in July, but the flood happened, another case of stuff not going to plan.

We didn't get a great deal of rain. It was only a constant drizzle for about three to four months. But when the water table was up, the water had nowhere to go and came out of the mountains much faster than I expected. With the amount of rain we had, I looked at it thinking, I've seen this before. It will come into the park and dissipate like it always does.

The day before the flood, I'd been having a beer at a mate's place. When I walked out, I said, 'Catch you tomorrow.'

When I got home, I thought I'd better have a look at the creek. I walked down a hundred or so metres. It was sitting at about six meters, still inside the bank. I returned to check it every now and then.

It was up to the March flood level, around 8.4 metres and maybe 10 to 15 metres off the back fence. That's nothing to worry about because it's still got quite a rise to get up to the yard. It was coming in and out a couple of inches at a time. I thought, yep, it's peaked.

I went back inside. I could still hear the water rushing through the grass in the front park.

Then I started checking on it hourly, and it didn't do much in the first couple of hours. It wasn't until maybe two or three in the morning that I went for one last look at it. I was quite confident it had peaked, but it had peaked higher.

I didn't realise this was the rush of all the different waters gathering together and coming down. It was about four o'clock in the morning. I still had to go to work the next day, but I thought it was all good, so I went to bed.

My alarm went off, and I thought I could hear something. As the water rose higher, it got into some longer grass, and I could hear it flattening it.

That was not good. It had risen about another two metres in about two hours. That was the biggest rush and rise I've ever seen in that river bed.

It had started coming in the back gate. I started running around, trying to save stuff in sheds. I went to the first shed that was beginning to take water, my main workshop, a 20-foot container.

I had a lot of very good tooling in that container. I collect vintage hobby lathes, some of which are pretty rare. I was running around in that shed but couldn't save anything.

I put stuff up as high as I could, shut the container, and stepped out into the water. When I reached the second shed, water was starting to enter it. Then, all three sheds were full of water.

My wife was still in bed. I woke her up and suggested she get a cup of coffee and a shower. She woke up bleary-eyed, looked at me, and said, 'No, it'll be fine.'

I said, 'You might want to take a look out the window.' The water was about 30 meters away, hitting the tar right out the front. She looked at it and still thought we'd be fine but went for her coffee and shower while I ran around trying to put stuff up high in the house.

It's hard. The water's coming, and you don't know where it will stop. I had an intuition, almost like something was helping me, so I put stuff at a certain height. Funnily enough, that's about the height at which it went through the house, about knee-deep.

Some of it was treasures; I got most of them. There was even a chest next to our bed. I don't know how I managed it, but I lifted it up onto the bed by myself. I moved so much stuff, but I'm not sure how I did it.

Certain things keep taking you back every time. Some of them are the sounds that trigger you. Even leading up to this discussion, I've started having dreams again. The other night, I was running around trying to save everything, and I couldn't because we were in a washing machine—even the car was in there. It's sights and sounds that trigger these things.

Sometimes, at night, I still hear the gurgling sound. When floodwaters come across the ground, they displace the air in there, so any air pockets get filled up, bubble out, and it's like the ground boils. I heard this come through the floor when I was running around the house trying to get stuff out.

The flood was knee-high, and you could hear it resonating as it approached the floorboards underneath. As it got to the floorboards, it was a weird sensation because it lifted the carpet and the material under it.

It became like walking on a trampoline, you're bouncing around on it. That boiling sound underneath the floor stayed with me for a long time. For six or eight months, I'd wake up hearing it in my sleep.

It's almost a feeling of panic. You can't describe it, but I'll do my best because people need to understand what it does to them in the long term. Now, if I smell a particular smell, like sewage, or I hear something, it puts me right back in there.

Your feeling of control is gone, and you're at the mercy of whatever's coming at you. With floods, you don't know where it's going to stop. It's hard, and sometimes it can put you in a pretty dark place again. Even just looking at some photos, I can almost describe what it smelled and sounded like at that particular time.

At one point, I walked into the laundry, which was lower than the rest of the floor in the house. It got inundated first, and there was a little crack in the concrete where there was some pipework underneath. All you could hear was the water displacing the air out of there. It was different from the bubbling that was coming out of the ground.

We were unsure what to do. Nobody is coming around handing you a brochure saying what you need to do. The first thing is to throw any canned goods or food in your cupboard. You can replace it. That's one of those things I tried to save, but two weeks after the flood, we found out that the house was badly contaminated with E. Coli, and we had been living in the house for about two weeks.

The only assistance we received was from some community people and a couple of stubborn mates who drove out to help. The area was shut down, and floods were happening all around.

The main road to town was still open, but it wouldn't be open for much longer. At this point, the only road open was the road into Singleton, but we heard it wasn't long before that road would be closed as well.

We didn't know what would happen to Singleton, so we camped on the roadside with the dog. She's not a real social dog, she usually lives in the lounge.

We had no communication to know what other people were doing apart from people stopping by. We saw no emergency services. We had nothing. We had no information besides this water is in our house now.

We were on the side of the road. We'd already saved what we could and been back into waist-deep water to push my old ute out and get my bike out of the house.

Believe it or not, our water delivery drivers were the only people who showed up to help. Those blokes went above and beyond. They went out into the paddock across the road, where there were horses on a mound in the middle of the paddock, which soon afterwards was totally surrounded by water.

Those blokes pulled up and went straight out into that paddock. They were neck-deep in water, leading horses. After they got the horses to safety up on the hill, they turned their attention to helping us. They were absolute champions. No one asked them to help. They just showed up and did it.

They are young local blokes, and they're renowned for their helpfulness. When something goes wrong, they're there to help. They even pestered us all night by coming back and making sure we were okay.

That's the community spirit that got us through it. I hate to say this, but I'd love to thank emergency services for what they did, but I can't. They didn't help us. We only saw people from emergency services two weeks after the flood. I jumped on Facebook and thanked the family and friends who came out and helped us.

One of my friends who was part of the Bulga Community Centre saw this, and the next thing we knew, we had help from everywhere. My phone was ringing, and people were showing up.

We still hadn't eaten properly. We were living on stuff like baked beans. All our supplies were all wet or gone. Even our medication was gone.

At 11 am the next day after the flood, the water was down to the floorboards again, so I went straight back in. As I opened the back screen door, suddenly, all this stuff started flowing out of the house.

Oh, there goes the shampoo and conditioner, our pills, and a piece of paper—it was a card to my wife perched up in the mesh of the screen. I'm also a drummer, so I have drumsticks everywhere.

I walked into the house thinking, this doesn't look too bad.

Then I was bucketing mud off stuff and wandering around without shoes. But it wasn't mud. It's not a good feeling to know what I was cleaning out. Of course, we realised it was contaminated, and everything was basically gone. We don't own this place, we have rented it for many years. We threw all our stuff out the front. We saved the bed and started ripping the carpet up.

Then, they sent out the EPA people who did the swab tests. That's when we found out about E. Coli. We had been working in a bio-contaminated site.

What happened next was not fun. We both ended up with stomach issues afterwards. It affected my wife more than me.

I was wet for weeks. I wore the same gum boots, I don't even think I had socks on. The first time I took the gum boots off was a mission because they were stuck on.

I had sores all over my body that wouldn't heal. They gave me a lot of antibiotics, which made me constipated, and I was also taking some quite hefty pain relief due to three fractured ribs that came about from moving stuff I shouldn't have. But they didn't pick up on that for a long time.

I spent an entire weekend by myself. I ripped the gearbox out of my car and rebuilt it on the bench out of three broken gearboxes because I had to move the car. I felt something tear in my groin. It's never been the same since; something's moved inside and doesn't work like before.

It was full-on physically, doing all this hard labour and trying to save things, only to realise that the whole site was contaminated. The positive side I tried to take from it was that there had been a lot of stuff I didn't know what to do with, including 90% of my dad's estate stuff.

When we found out the actual. E. coli results showed animal faecal matter, including from chickens. We only have a dog. That's when we started reassessing everything else.

Once that happened, at about the two-week mark, we began what became known as the 'Road to Nowhere Tour', which consisted of my nightly updates on social media for family and friends just to let everybody know we were okay after a couple of weeks.

My phone rang off its choppers. I couldn't answer it because everything was wet. We were trying to dry stuff, but it just kept raining. We were living in a glorified camper trailer, which became known as the tent on wheels.

So, the three of us lived there for two weeks, and I worked around the clock. The poor old dog followed me around everywhere, like a bad smell.

Apparently, we all smelled bad.

At the end of the first month, they found Carina and the dog emergency accommodation in a boarded-up farmhouse about 15 kilometres away. The journey into the farmhouse was very rough.

The old boarded-up farmhouse was full of rodents, snakes, and bandicoots. I used to sit on the veranda up there, shooting the rats with the slug gun; it's quite a humane way to do it.

One night, I think it was the first or second night, Carina stayed up at the farm by herself, glad to have a bed, roof, floor, and fireplace. I was getting there about 11:30 pm. I thought I'd better go back to the tent where I was now illegally squatting. The ute bogged straight down to the chassis, and that's where it stayed for the night. I tried to get the ute out and thought I had to walk and go to work tomorrow.

I walked back out of the farmhouse covered in mud so we went and tried to get it out again. Still couldn't get it out. I said, 'Something's telling me I've got to walk.'

People were going around stealing things, so I had to get back there for security purposes. I got a lift back from someone working for mine security, and luckily, I had another car to get to work the next day.

But the ute had to be pushed out with an excavator. That became my nightly routine. Every night, I would pull up at what I was calling home, a glorified tent on wheels.

I even had some mates call in one night. For some reason, they didn't hang around too long. I was a bit feral-looking; I smelled bad and wasn't overly friendly to anybody. I had my personal rubbish going on from what had happened to us.

These dudes stuck around for about five or ten minutes. I jokingly said, 'Go on, piss off then, you blokes are just jealous of how I'm living.' We all had a laugh, and off they went.

I tried to hide much of what was really going on with humour. It doesn't work. It got me.

Carina was living out in the bush. Although we had been married for many years, we hadn't spent much time apart, and this was a big learning curve for me. I had to fend for myself, although we had a lot of support from the neighbours, who fed us quite well for some time.

I wasn't in a good place. I possibly went full-blown nuts to a degree. I still had common sense and didn't do anything too stupid. I only bought one motorcycle because I thought I needed it to get in and out of the farm in case the ute wouldn't get in and out of there.

I went back to save some stuff. But most of what I saved wasn't even mine. I saved a bit of Dad's stuff and a few good things.

Then, we were told we could not re-enter the house as the lease was now null and void. We're basically homeless. I didn't think I'd get to almost 50 and be a homeless person who still had a decent job.

After the initial swab results, they said, 'You're out, you cannot enter that premises.' They'd let us go in there for about an hour at a time with strict conditions and only to get our stuff out.

When we became homeless a month after the flood, one of the real estate chiefs said, 'It's going to take you at least two years to get back on your feet after this.'

I laughed at her, saying, 'No, she'll be right. I'll be back on my feet in six months. It'll be fine.' Wasn't she right?

This is a process. It takes a lot of time, especially when you are stubborn and don't accept anybody's help. I wanted help, but I didn't. When people came to me and asked what I wanted them to do, I'd say, 'I don't know.' How do you accept help from somebody when you don't know what you need to do? I felt like I was running around bumping into brick walls.

I was being impacted by the stress of the whole thing, the flood.

But it's the last thing on your mind. What came to my mind when that water started coming into that house was that we've got to get out of here and save ourselves because nobody's coming to do it for us.

Carina has told me numerous times that if I had not been home, she would have waited for emergency services before leaving the house.

We had bushfires in 2017-2018, which also took a toll because we're constantly on bushfire watch. We saw the Rural Fire Service regularly. They would regularly drive by and check up on the community, looking at the fuel on the ground. They even came and slashed particular areas as a preventative measure.

We saw nothing like that this time, and it's a shame because prior to this, in the 2007 floods, we had the SES come around and say, 'The flood is going to do this. It's going to do that.'

I said, 'Look, it's all cool. We've got a hill behind us. If anything goes wrong, we're going straight up there and not worrying about anything.'

2007 was a slow flood that reached roughly nine meters at home. It was quite a substantial flood that hung around for a long time. The water sat in the park for days.

This one came in and out so quickly. The sheer speed even caught the emergency services off guard. They say they like to listen to local knowledge. If it had stuck at what I predicted, the water would have entered our yard but not the house.

Unfortunately, it went about a metre higher than I predicted. Their data was incorrect, saying it went to 11.1 meters, but that is when the data stopped reading because the monitor went underwater.

From my measurements using the 2007 datapoint on the bridge, where the high tide was in 2022, it reached around 11.4 -11.5 metres.

I can never repay people for how they helped us out. The places you go after in your own head while you're battling this thing: firstly, the panic and shock of it.

Just keep yourself going. You don't take in what's going on around you. Even now, when I look at some of these photos and realise we lost all that, you can still have moments where you've got to go and sit down.

When I tried to return to work, I had lost all my social skills. I couldn't speak to people, so I spent a lot of time in that tent by myself. Sometimes, the battle was just making a cup of tea. Other times, the battle was lying down because of the pain from my broken and worn-out body.

Then I'd try and sleep, but I couldn't sleep. I ended up taking a lot of Valium and painkillers to try to shut my brain off. That didn't work.

Then, there are some of the inappropriate things people say. I was telling somebody about what had happened afterwards, and somebody I knew had overheard it.

They said, 'Oh, get over it. We're sick of hearing about it.' That's really not appropriate, but I bit my tongue.

One of the kindest things someone did for me happened one day when I was sitting down and having a moment. I was sitting out the back on a step at work, my body in agony, I was 200 per cent exhausted, and there was water coming out of my eyes. It must have been raining!

One of my co-workers, who I've worked with for many years, sat down beside me, popped his hand on my shoulder, and just sat there. That is the kind of help and support people need, not advice.

It was the simple act of just sitting there with me, knowing you're not alone. He's had his own issues with life as well. Nobody gets it easy. We all have issues. It's how you work through them that makes a difference. He walked inside and walked back out where I was sitting, and he handed me a card.

He said, 'If you want to talk to someone, mate, ring this bloke.'

I did. Because I'm a bloke, I thought I was tough enough to deal with and hide it. All I did was hide what was really going on.

I mentioned changing what I would tell people when they'd ask about how we went.

After seeing the look on their face, I had to change what I was saying from, 'We lost just about everything we own,' to, 'It's okay. We saved a few good things.'

But I was lying.

Yes, we managed to save a few good things, like all the trinkets on the top shelf, but we no longer have a top shelf to put them on. We still have stuff boxed up, but we don't know if it will ever come out of those boxes. I've got sheds of musical instruments, but I don't know if they're okay.

Two years down the track, I'm still cleaning things up, pulling things apart, and trying to fix and put them back together. If it doesn't work, I throw it out. I thought I could save everything, and I can't.

There comes a time when you've just got to go bugger it, it's gone. Some of the stuff that we threw out was quite substantial, and some of it was not.

It's the little things, like our son recently visiting. We were sitting around at night talking about young people's handwriting.

One of us said, your handwriting was pretty good. I don't know if it was me or Carina. He said, 'No, my handwriting is terrible.' I reached onto the shelving in one of the rooms and pulled out his first kindergarten handwriting book. He's in his mid-to-late twenties now, and that got him a little bit. He wasn't here through the flood event, but he's also lost stuff. A lot of his childhood memories were there.

That's when you go through that entire loss all over again. It's not just that one little item, everything comes back. 'Oh shit, this is the situation I'm in. And I'm still in that situation now.'

I've got cars and bikes to fix up. I'm still trying to save tooling. Most of it just stayed in the shed because we were in survival mode, though we did what we could. The future for now is to keep trying to save what I can and throw out what I can't.

It's certainly changed my outlook on life. A lot of things I used to think were important now are not. Hopefully, the future for us is to get through the other side of this, whenever that is.

We don't know when that will be because we're still going through it.

Some of the things people have done to help us through this have been mind-blowingly awesome. I can't thank them enough.

If people want to help, the help has to be appropriate. Sometimes, it's not. Some people can hinder, and some people can help.

Unfortunately, the short-term goal for me with this situation is to try to raise awareness of many of these issues regarding why people like us were forgotten.

I've used that as a driver to push through and mask a little of what I really feel. There are times when I get exhausted, and it is overwhelming, and I must stop.

It was over 12 months before I even stopped. I just kept going. I'd finish work, then go home and work, then I'd sleep for an hour or two and then go to work, then go home and work.

That's all it was. It was just constant; it didn't stop. There was always something to do, and there's still always something to do now.

At the moment, I'm trying to save tooling. Flood water carries not only contaminants but is also quite corrosive due to its electrolytic value.

One of the things that got saved was my dad's drum kit, which meant a lot to me. I would have lost it if the water had gone an inch higher.

At the moment, I believe surviving is the key to this. I don't consider myself a victim of a natural disaster. I'm a survivor, and I'll push through and do whatever I need to do.

That's how I've gone through this whole journey. The 'Road to Nowhere Tour' has been about getting to the end, but honestly, I can't see the end of it. There's always something else I've got to do.

Our place looks nice now. It's got all new carpet and is freshly painted. It's come up really well. It took 9-10 months to get to that stage, and they did a great job. For a long time, that did not feel like home. It still doesn't, yet it does. It's the oddest feeling.

It carries a fair deal of sentiment to me because we've had a lot of life experience there. Yes, it's still home, but we know this area and what can happen now. Historically, there have been floods through there before. Maybe higher, but I'm not sure how accurate the data is.

When I see flooding elsewhere, I want to help those people. I want to say. 'It's okay. You'll get through this.' My thoughts are with all those people. I know what it's like. I've been through it. There is a way out, but it takes its toll.

What I'm doing now is trying to help others. Being blokes, we all try to power through, but that doesn't always help. I hid much of what was going on with a sense of humour and by not telling people what was happening.

Many people have called me a hero because of what we have survived. I'm not, I'm just an average bloke who did what he had to do to get through it.

I believe anybody would do the same to get through to the other side.

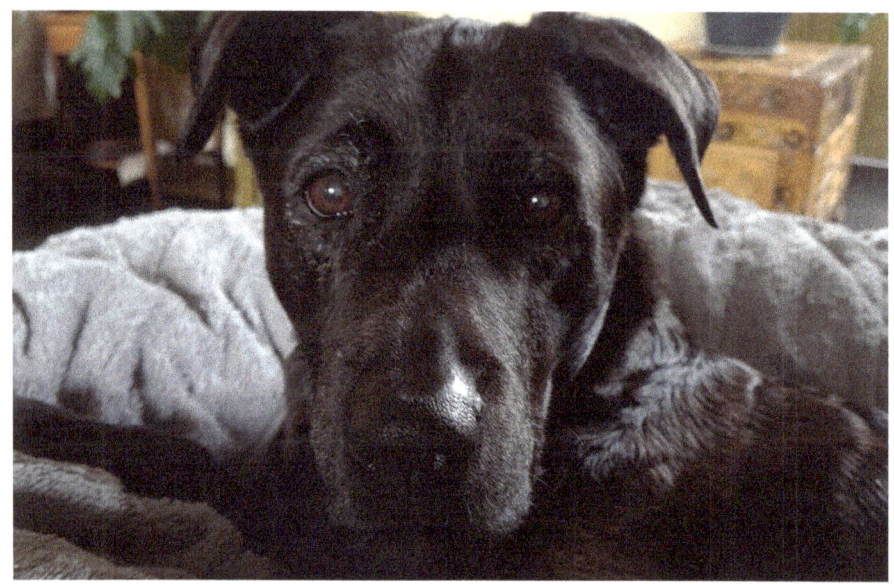

Jess is a beloved Mooen Family member.

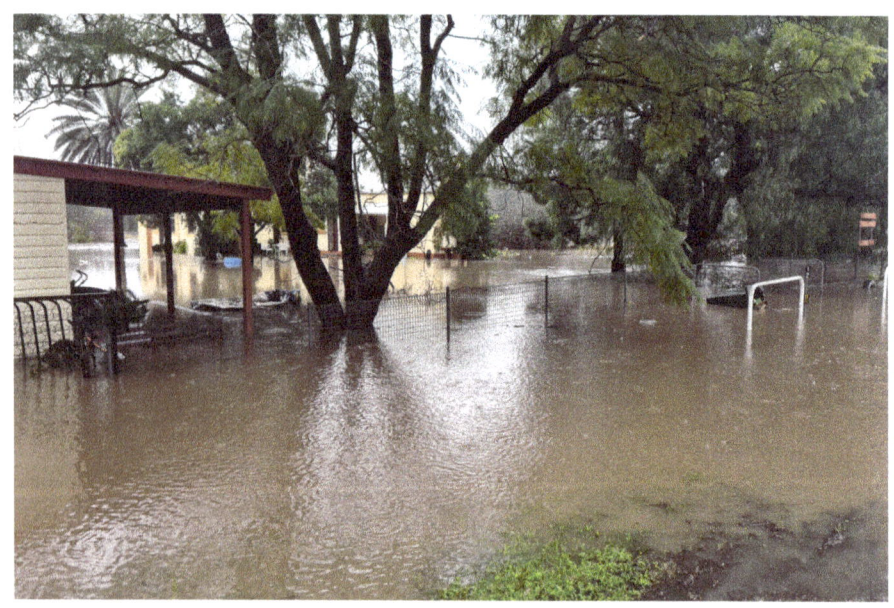

The Moonen Family home at Warkworth.

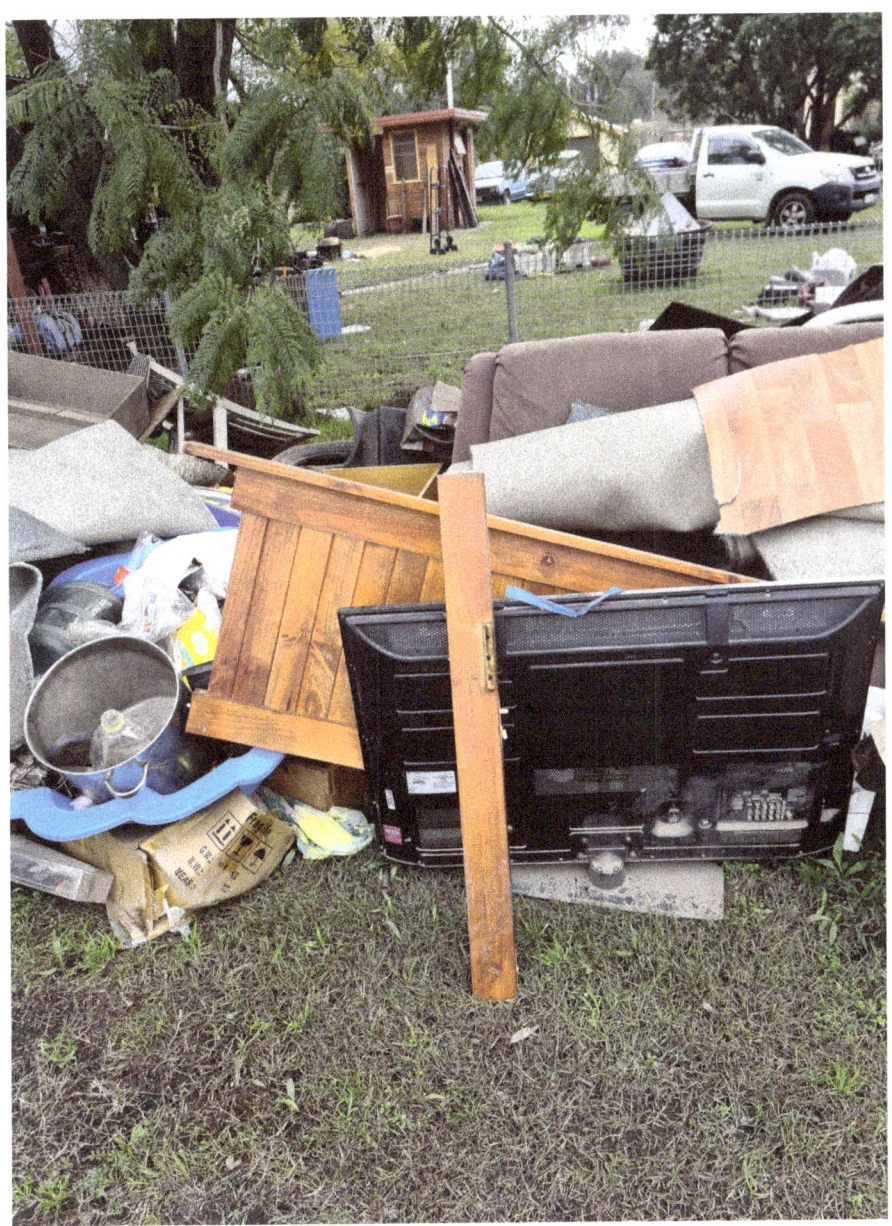

Bottom Personal Belongings waiting for collection

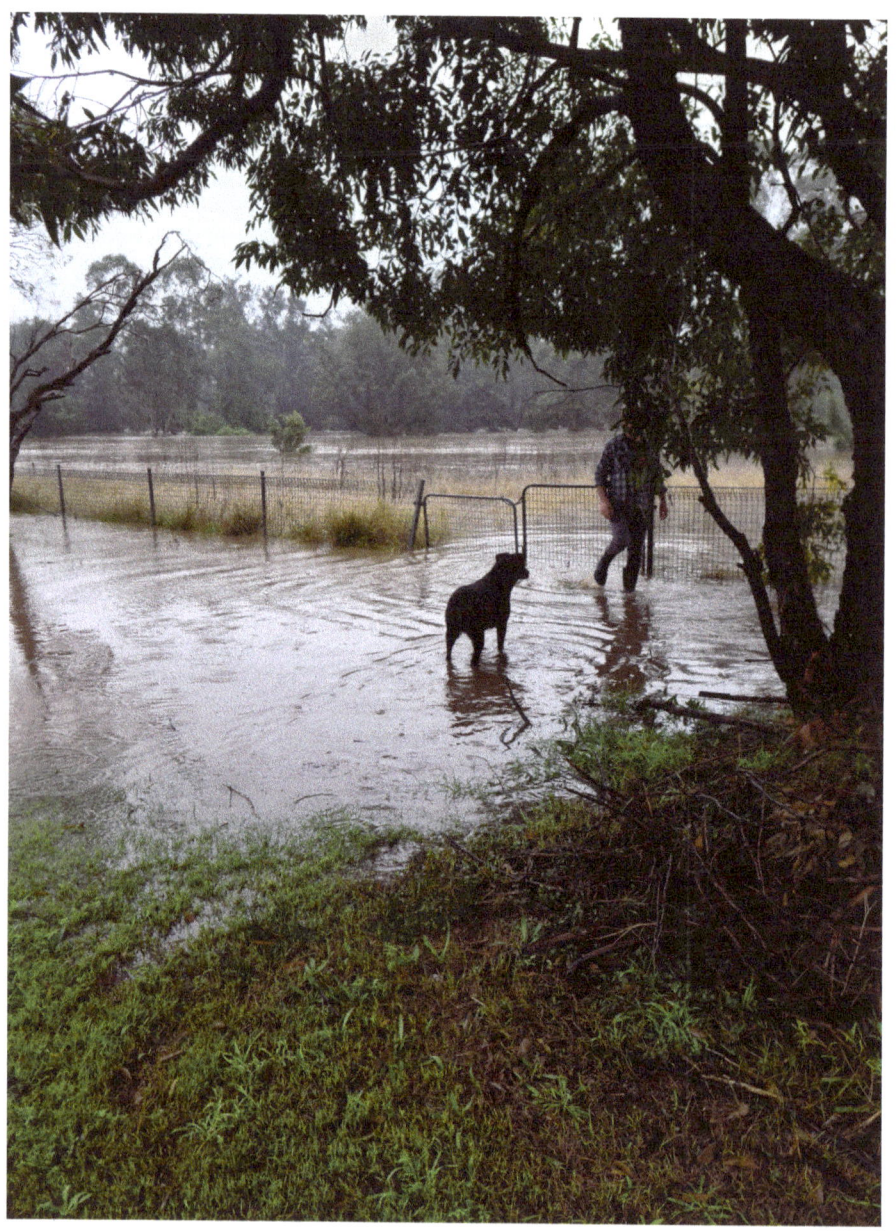

Leith with Jess at Warkworth

LEITH MOONEN

CARINA MOONEN

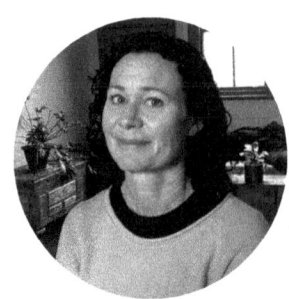

Carina and her husband Leith were severely impacted by the 2022 flood. Because they live at Warkworth, away from the main flood area and were cut off by flooded roads, they were not assisted by emergency services.

'I was a little bit bitter that nobody had come, simply because if Leith hadn't been here, I would not have left. I would have waited for someone to come and save me. The dog and I would have been on my bed because that's the highest point and there was literally no one coming for us.'

'In the future, I want them not to forget the little people. The alerts had come through Bulga, Broke, and Singleton. For some reason, I thought that because Warkworth wasn't named, we must be OK. It's a silly attitude, but it is what it is.'

Her husband Leith has also shared his story and both together offer us a devastating picture of what they went through. The ordeal is still not over for them.

Carina's story is raw and very honest, but like the other Kintsugi Heroes we have spoken to she expressed her gratitude at the many acts of generosity and kindness from members of the community

Prior to July 5th, 2022, we were a standard bunch of people. Leith and I have always worked. I was an educator at a preschool for 16 years and was in early intervention before that. We'd had a few dramas leading up to the flood, but we were regular people cruising along, living our lives.

We live in a very old school at Warkworth. We moved to Warkworth when my son was 18 months old, and he's 27 this year. It's such a great spot. My husband plays the drums, so nobody wants to live too close to us. We've got the river behind us, dogs, and an only child. I always had pets. It's a beautiful spot. Our closest neighbour is the coal mine. They make as much noise as we do, so it works out perfectly.

We were used to floods. The water spilled over into the park in front of us numerous times over the years. It was entertaining because there were days off school, and we couldn't go to work. We'd hang out as a family, watch the water come up, and then watch the water go down.

I've never considered that we would flood.

I had gone to bed the night before, very blasé saying, 'We've been here for over 20 years. It's come up into the park. Never had to worry.' Leith was keeping an eye on it, but honestly, I thought he was making a fuss about nothing.

Then he woke me up and said, 'I think you should get up. I think this might be something.'

I still scoffed at him, tidied up a bit, and Leith said, 'You probably should pack a bag. You need to go.' That was when I looked out the front steps and thought, oh, it is actually coming quite up. It came around us, which I wasn't expecting.

I clearly didn't take it seriously because the bag I packed had a book and a spare book just in case, a pillow, a blanket, my medication and my handbag. I grabbed the dog, and as I went off the top step, the dog baulked, and I thought, we'll be fine, this is what we're doing. I stepped off the top step into the water. It was above my knees, and I hadn't considered how cold the water would be and how much of a push it would have.

Out the front of our house, we've got a big concrete slab, then a concrete path. We'll be fine as long as I keep to the path. Off we went. The dog's all about swimming. She was not very happy, and I stepped off the path, so I dropped down about that much. That was when I felt the pull of the water. I wasn't panicking, but I was a little bit, oh, this is something.

I got put up on the side of the road and still didn't think much of it. There are people here getting both cars and everything out. My car was out, and I continued to take photos. I had a joke. I didn't take it too seriously.

Then I saw that it had come in through the lounge room, which was the highest point. That was my last photo. That was when I left, and that's when things changed.

Before I'd left, Leith had said to me, you should probably get yourself organised, and I had replied, 'We don't need to worry; someone will come and tell us what to do.' I had complete faith in emergency services. Somebody would come and either get us out or give us some information.

But nobody came, whereas when we went through the fires, which were a distance from us, the RFS called in and said be prepared. I was above and beyond prepared for the fires. Cars packed, houses packed, everything's organised. This time, I didn't even take a phone charger. Because I thought somebody would come and tell me what to do.

We moved up onto the hill on the side of the road with the cars. I didn't even take a spare pair of shoes. As soon as I put my shoes on, I stepped into the water. I had wet feet for God knows how long, and that was it. We slept in the car, and as soon as the water dropped the next day, we came in, and it wasn't very good. It was knee-high all the way through the house.

We focused on the house itself. Leith and another bloke were pulling up carpets and other stuff, and I was looking around because you keep all your child's things through their schooling and all the rest of it. It was all underneath the bed, and it was all ruined.

Everything I kept from my only child was destroyed. His baby book, photos, books, things that meant nothing to other people. For me, they were irreplaceable.

That was very upsetting, but then you've got a variety of people coming onto the property saying, 'What do you want us to do?'

I was saying, 'I've got no clue.' It was still raining. We're trying to save things, but you couldn't get dry. You couldn't do anything about them.

We stayed here for two weeks, then Leith said, 'We can't stay in the house anymore. We're homeless.'

I didn't love that idea, so we borrowed a camper trailer from his auntie and popped it out the front. The dog was too old and fat to get onto the bed, and my back was too bad, so the dog and I camped for a couple of weeks on an air mattress on the camper trailer floor. That was bloody cold.

About a week after the flood, I got a stomach bug, so I was camping with a stomach bug in the middle of winter, trying not to complain. There was no point whinging. The real estate agent was trying to organise me somewhere to go to get me off the property. We found a house in the middle of nowhere, and I said, 'It's fine.' The real estate agent and the coal mine helped us out.

After we had been in the camper trailer for two weeks, the house up on the hill was ready. Leith said, 'When you're ready to go, go.'

I said, 'No, I'll stay with you.' Then I got too sick and ended up saying, 'You've got to get me out of here.'

Leith drove me to the house at night and dropped me off there. It was a house on a hill in the middle of nothing—no people, no cars, nothing. I said, 'We'll be fine. It's me and the dog; we'll be good.' As Leith left, he became bogged up to the axles in the driveway.

I was supposed to be up there for three months, 12 weeks. Everyone said, '12 weeks, you'll be fine.' I couldn't take my car up there.

I said, 'Yep, that'll be fine.' I've never lived alone before. I moved out here in August and didn't move back until March.

The floodwaters were not clean river water; it was not mud we were playing with. But I had no clue about what to do. The old people say, 'Clean everything up, everything, give it a clean, it'll be fine.' Which is true in some cases. But our whole septic had gone through the house, not only our septic. It was everything from downstream.

I had a stomach bug for three months, and once I was up on that hill, there was no coming down. There was no going to the doctor, though I could go to the dentist. There were rats, snakes, bees, and more wildlife.

We were outside the operational zone, so we weren't updated. It was like we didn't exist. Then, all of a sudden, word must have spread, and we started to get the army, the fireys, and various people. It was a lot to deal with because they asked me, 'What do you want me to do?'

I'd say, 'I have got no clue. I don't know.'

It started raining again recently, and we are supposed to get a lot of rain in the next couple of days. But I knew the chances of that much water again were slim. However, I walked around the house yesterday and thought, what would I do? I don't think I could start over again. I think I would walk away.

What changed for me was that people's perception of it upset me. They would say it's only stuff; everything's replaceable. Some things are not. What sticks in my mind the most is that we had to put everything out in front for the council to come and clean up.

I happened to be home when the council came to take that stuff away, and the sound of the breaking glass as they scooped everything up to put it in the garbage stuck in my mind because it was not rubbish. That was my entire life.

It's sickening to the bottom of your stomach to pile up your life in front of your house. You're throwing away photos because they are all those precious things you hang on to, and I'm very sentimental. I am that person who has kept every single card that I have ever been given in my entire life.

Preschool photos, all of the birthday cards and Christmas cards that your children make you. I keep all that stuff. Our little dog had passed away not long before the flood. I had taken prints from my dog because we were all going to get them tattooed. That's gone, too.

Although these might be small things to people and not valuable, to me, throwing away my son's baby book was heart breaking.

I ended up not feeling I could keep going. I was there trying to help Leith, not realising that, because he's still going to work, I'm here through the day by myself. I didn't realise he would worry about how I was feeling and going. It reached the point where Leith said, and he meant no harm from it, 'It's not that you're useless, it's that you're not very useful.'

He was worrying about me, so I decided it was best to go up the hill and get out of everyone's way. That's what I did.

Initially, it worked for me. I needed to escape this situation. I was getting more and more ill. I was tired, my back hurt and all the rest of it. The dog was not coping, and she started to have a go at people.

It wasn't a good situation. It ended up being the most stunning solitary confinement I could imagine. I was up there for 23 hours a day by myself and saw Leith for an hour or two. Most of that was to have a quick meal, and he would sleep because he was still living in the camper trailer, trying to work, and coming up to bring me food.

After a while, you forget how to interact with people. These things change people's personalities. It changed the dynamic of my marriage a little bit. Leith and I have always been at 50:50 in decision-making. We both worked. I don't work at the moment. It went from that to Leith making the decisions on my behalf, some of which were bad decisions. Some of them were not so bad.

Coming back has been a challenge. I'm not quite sure how I fit back into things as yet. The problem is that it's coming up to two years, it'll be two years in July. I had always planned to stay here until we won the lotto and then retire to the beach. Now, I'm not quite so sure. It's a big thing. When you're moving to a home with your family, my son had his bedroom and all that sort of thing. All of that's gone now, so it's different.

Something that's changed for me since the flood is the local community. When we were up on the side of the road, I met all of my neighbours. I had not met them previously other than a wave as I drove down the road because that's the country thing, but I had never really met them. Some of them would come to see how we were getting on while we were on the hill.

A little while after that, our neighbours up on the hill came down to see how we were. I had no shoes, and all of my shoes and clothes were destroyed. I was left with the clothes on my back, which I'd been sleeping in for the last couple of days.

I had a random pair of boots that I found somewhere. No shampoo or conditioner, all of that stuff's gone. Although they're tiny things, they're important things. When the neighbour came down, she looked at me, then went back home and came back with some money and said, 'Please go and buy yourself some boots.'

I was initially mortified because we don't ask for help or take charity or anything like that. It was a big thing, instead of saying, 'No, I'm fine. I'll wander around in thongs.' I had to say, 'Thank you so much, I appreciate that.'

Since then, we've become very firm friends with the neighbours. They helped us and fed us for quite a while, which was incredibly kind.

The government offered grants, so we had to go to Bulga and walk into a room with other people like us. You're entitled to this money from the government.

It was horrendous. I was embarrassed and ashamed that we were in this position and would need assistance from the outside. You have to go through hoops, finding your worst flood photos to show them, and of course, they wouldn't transfer, or this wouldn't happen, or that wouldn't happen. You're going back through these photos over and over again, and it was awful.

I understand why they have to make it so difficult because I understand that there are people out there who would take advantage of the situation. The people who work in Service NSW or whatever it is must have some feel for the people that they're literally face to face with. I don't know how they would go about it. Still, there needs to be a better system because it's bad enough being there and having to ask for help, let alone going over and over it again.

I was a bit bitter that nobody had come, simply because I would not have left if Leith hadn't been here. I would have waited for someone to come and save me. The dog and I would have been on my bed because that was the highest point, and no one was coming for us.

In the future, I want them not to forget the little people. The alerts had come through Bulga, Broke, and Singleton. For some reason, I thought that because Warkworth wasn't named, we must be OK. It's a silly attitude, but it is what it is. With the flood alerts that are on now, it's still the same, so in my mind, I'm thinking, it'll be fine.

I must admit, I am much more anxious when it rains now. I've always loved the rain, but now it's in the back of my mind because, after the flood, many people came to the house and said, 'It's happened once within a five-year period, chances are it's going to happen again.'

Since the flood, I have learned that I am stronger than I thought, not physically but mentally. I am now absolutely petrified of snakes. That was a new thing. I'm a country girl, so I've always said snakes are more scared of you than you are of them. No one is more scared than me of the king browns I had up there.

I also learnt that you have to have a buddy and keep that buddy close because you can't do it alone. What Leith and I worked out separately is that as much use as we are on our own, together, we can make it.

Although he doesn't bloody listen when somebody tells him to slow down and chill out, he loves and adores me and the dog. The number of times I would say to him, 'Don't drive up here after work, it's late, it's raining, you're tired, we're fine', he would still show up in that ute. He'd put wood, food, and water into a wheelbarrow and barrow that up to me through the mud so we could light the fire and have something to eat. I admire Leith.

But in the long term, it's always going to be in the back of our minds that this could happen again, and it could be worse. At the same time, I think of people who have been in the Lismore floods—that was worse than our situation, but I think loss is loss.

I have learned that everyone's perception about what you should do, or what they would do, is different from what actually happens. You can go into it with the best plan in the world. We all know how the best-laid plans in life work.

The best thing that has happened to us since the flood is that we've made some lifelong friends.

If a natural disaster can't destroy a perfectly good marriage, then I don't think anything can. Sometimes, you're stronger than you think. Even if you're feeling weak and useless at the time, you're still bringing something to the party, even if it's something small.

What am I grateful for now? I've always worked, but for the last few years,

I've not been working, and my days are quite long. I am incredibly grateful for my big boof-head dog, who has not left my side since we stepped off into the flipping water, and Leith. He was incredible and continues to be.

That is what I'd be grateful for.

Based on my experiences, I'd like to share that you should stick with your people. They're the ones who will look after you, even if they're idiots at the time.

If there's another flood, I'll be heading straight up the hill!

MICK MCARDLE

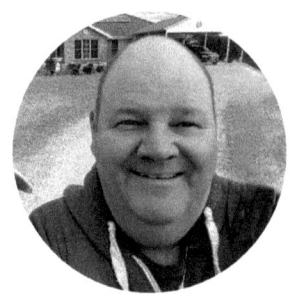

Mick McCardle is a man who was acknowledged by the village as being an absolute hero when it came to supporting the community. His role was essential and his heart was huge.

Born in 1963, he was in the ADF from 1981 to 2013. He currently owns a small business. He was the Singleton Citizen of the year for 2023 and is the president of the Broke Residents Community Association.

Mick's story is about his personal experience of the catastrophic 2022 flood, as well as sharing the story of being in charge of the operations centre at the Broke Community Hall during the flood.

'Because of my 30-odd years in the military, mainly overseas in operations, I came into the job to head up the operations centre because I knew what was involved and that when I was down there at the hall, I had to portray, okay, this is what we've got to do and get it done.'

I joined the army after working as a kitchen hand at King's School in 1980. I had lost my job there. I can't remember why, but my dad came into my bedroom and said, 'Sign this.'

Back then, you could sign up for three or six years. I thought, 'I'm going to sign for three years.' I did 22 years of regular army and 10 years of reserve army. It was the best thing that I ever did.

The majority of my time in the army was spent in logistics. I did an eight-month tour in Africa with what they call UNTAG, the United Nations Treaty Assistance Group in Namibia. I learned so much about what you hold dear in Australia when you see other countries, especially countries like that, which are pretty poor.

Coming back from there, I continued with logistics. I began to get command positions like Squadron Sergeant Major. I was second in command there at one stage. That's how I finished off my career. It was a good experience because you had a fair-sized group of blokes that you had to administer and control.

My wife and I moved here to Broke in 2016. We wanted a tree change from suburbia. We live right on the edge of Broke Village.

Leading up to July 6th, 2022, it had rained a few days beforehand. We were caught in our street because floodwaters diverted from the brook, went between and around the backs of houses, and overflowed over our street. We were stuck here for two days before the floodwaters started receding enough that we could get out.

When the floodwaters receded enough, I went into Broke to find Kathleen, the fire captain. I saw her at Broke Hall, where they were setting up an emergency area and flood command centre.

When I saw Kathleen, I asked, 'Is there anything I can do?' She was shattered. She'd probably done the best part of 48 hours straight because of her role with the Rural Fire Service.

She said, 'Can you take this over? Can you run with this?'

I didn't give it a second thought; I said, 'Yep, I'll do that.' I got stuck there for another 14 days.

The funny thing was that where I live, because we got cut off from the village, we were in a bubble. None of the surrounding properties had any floodwaters in them.

Another couple of places were the same, so when I got out and drove down to the Broke Hall, it was an eye-opener. I couldn't believe how much water had come through the town.

Then, when I got into the operations centre, the first day I got in, we were working with only one whiteboard. By the end of it, we had about 12.

It was just the extent of how much this had impacted the Wollombi area, from Payne's Crossing up to us at Broke and then out to Fordwich and Bulga, that put in perspective how big this was.

The way the floodwaters rose surprised many people, even the SES. I remember them coming down our street to say, 'You're going to have a look at evacuating soon.' When I walked with them out to the front of my place to the street, they said, 'You've got to go now.'

It was starting to come over the road, and within an hour, it was coming over so fast you couldn't get out. Where it came over our road, it was the watercourse that took out Broke Road north of Broke, and it was amazing.

I remember the 2015 floods because I was in the army at Singleton Range. We had to leave there and go back to Adamstown in Newcastle.

When I talk to people after the floods of 2022, 2015 wasn't as bad. It hadn't flooded in the village for 50 years. I think it caught a lot of people off-guard. You don't expect it. It was definitely an eye-opener.

Because of my 30-odd years in the military, mainly overseas in operations, I came into the job to head up the operations centre because I knew what was involved and that when I was down there at the hall, I had to portray, okay, this is what we've got to do and get it done.

Luckily, we had support from many people, including Bulga Coal. The police, RFS, SES, and the army sent people out. We had people coming up from RFS Victoria and SES Victoria. The number of people that we had was incredible.

The situation in Broke reminded me a little of my overseas service. I remember one day seeing people come in and how distraught they were, and it took me back. But a cup of tea or coffee, a biscuit, and a chat with them perked them up.

The people who were helping me were probably some of the best people I've met, most of them locals. Some people from the council, the SES, and Services NSW, would occasionally drop in.

One of the biggest things that we had to address was the lack of water. When the floodwaters broke across Broke Road, north of Broke Road, it took out the main supply of water, and it took them about five days to get that reconnected.

Also, because Broke is on septic in the village, that situation needed to be sorted out.

I got in there a couple of days after the floods had receded, and they'd already started pumping out septic systems. It was just a matter of keeping track of it and making sure it happened.

The RFS were spraying out and getting mud out of garages, and we had what they call erosion holes under houses. No one had seen this phenomenon before, and it was because of the amount of water and how fast it was running. It would create erosion holes where people have stumps in their yards, like fence post stumps. There'd be a hole around them where the water had come in and pulled out all the dirt and taken it elsewhere.

There was also fixing roads and dealing with rubbish, so there was a lot of liaising with Stirling Council to get that sort of thing sorted out.

Where we live, we've got tank water, had no problems and were cooking off gas in about day two of the floods. My mate next door—Rob Disher—and I had a couple of generators floated in, so we were sweet.

We didn't know how high the water would rise. When it was peaking at two, three, and four o'clock in the morning, I began going down the back and checking the water levels to see where it was coming from. Luckily, it didn't come onto our property. We worked it out that if our place had flooded, Broke would have gone under by at least two and a half meters.

A mate of mine said it was a perfect storm because of where it was coming from, but we were also very lucky that there was no water coming into the Hunter River from the Patterson because that would have blocked everything up from moving north.

It was just freak storms. We were fortunate we never lost anyone. There were a couple of issues with a woman and her child getting stuck on the bridge. The SES and RFS had to evacuate them off the bridge, and then another guy got sucked under his house, but fortunately, he was spat out the other side.

I had to switch off from the human issues around me to a certain point. I know that when I started thinking about the human side of it, I'd have to walk away because I was getting upset. I remember quite clearly one morning when I was having a shower before I went back down to the hall. I was in the foetal position in my shower, crying.

It's hard to think about it now, but back then, it was 'Pull your bloody pants up, mate, get down there, do your job, and do it well.'

This event really pulled the community together. People came up to me saying, 'That old man hasn't spoken to his neighbours in 15 years, and yet now they're having a beer, and they're talking, and they're helping each other.'

It brought people together, and people helped each other. We'd have people come down to the operations centre saying, 'What can we do?'

Because we had so much support from other agencies, we said, go back to your place, go to your neighbours; if you can help them, please do. That's what they did. Everyone was happy with that.

To help and support people, we ran a shop down there, so if people needed a couple of rolls of toilet paper, hand sanitiser, food, women's toiletries, etc.— this was during COVID, and we had a few people with COVID around the same time.

The people would come in, and we'd say, 'All right, are you going to have a coffee there? Come on out, grab some stuff, and take it back home. Look after yourself.'

We had the GoFundMe page, so we gave people vouchers and cards so they could go shopping and get back to a little bit of normality. You can't pamper them too much. You've got to say, 'You're doing well, safe, and alive. Here are some tools for you to use to get back on track.'

We had counsellors and priests out there, and another mob was involved. They said they couldn't believe how fast we got into action compared to Lismore.

I don't know how it was in Lismore, but they were in awe. I'd tell them, 'We've got a great council that came straight out, and if I asked for something, I got it.' We had Bulga Coal, which did a hell of a lot about ballast and all that sort of stuff.

When houses were affected by these erosion holes, we had to fill them with ballast; otherwise, we would have lost them. It was one of those times when everyone pulled together, and it was amazing to see.

It was mentioned to me a few times that one of the things people liked about how I handled the situation was that I would give town meetings every couple of days. I'd bring everyone up to date on what's happening, what we've done, how things are happening, and our plans.

By our second town meeting, I was getting no questions, and everyone got the answers they needed.

People said the best thing that happened was that they were informed about what was happening and took solace from it. To me, that was one of the proudest things that we did, and again, that goes back to my army training about keeping people informed.

I've been greatly appreciated for how I handled the situation, which makes me feel very humble in some ways because of the number of other people who helped me along the way, including my wife. She couldn't get to work because of the floodwaters, but she was there helping us out in the hall and other community members.

When I received that Citizen of the Year award, it wasn't just for me. It was for everyone in Broke.

I think the community learned that it has come out of this with more situational awareness, so when we do get rain, as we're having at the moment, we can keep an eye on things.

People are more aware of what's going on regarding weather patterns and all that. You go back to two and a half years before when we had the fires; it was crazy. We had fires pretty much all around us. We've had a drought, mice, fire, COVID, and then floods. Give us a break, but everyone's pretty resilient. They continue on, pick up their big girl's pants, and keep going. I didn't say that to people because I didn't want to offend people. But that saying goes back to my army days: come on, get up, keep going.

The counsellors, priests, and chaplains were good because they kept an eye on people when we couldn't. The teams would come back from areas, and if someone was struggling, they'd let us know, and we'd go and chat with them.

That pulls many people back to the early days. They didn't know what would happen, and they didn't even know if their houses would be covered by insurance.

People can be ready for the next event to a certain extent. Many of us think it won't happen again in my lifetime, touch wood. I think many people in their own properties are more aware now that floods are here, and if it's going to flood again, I need to do this or that.

There were stories that came out of floods and one of them I remember is a couple trying to move horses. They nearly didn't get out because of how fast the water was going; it could have been much more serious. With awareness of the floodwaters and how fast they can rise, people know what they've got to plan for and are more confident that they can do what they can do.

As a logistics person, if we went through that sort of scenario again, I told the council that they need a 20-foot container with, tables, whiteboards, chairs, stationery, laptops, whatever, even if it sits at Singleton. They can deploy wherever within the LGA so that evacuation centres and operation centres can be set up within a moment's notice.

If a similar flood happened I probably would go straight down there, but I've also got my family to consider. Luckily my wife wasn't at work at the time of the floods.

She was on night shift, so she woke up and I told her 'You're not going anywhere, unless you've got a high-speed boat to get across the road.'

We discussed it when they came and saw us about evacuating my wife, Min, but we couldn't go because of the animals. We've got three dogs, two cats, and chickens. I don't think our biggest dog, a Rhodesian Ridgeback, would have been happy getting in a tinny to cross a raging river.

You do what you've got to do with animals as well. The thought of us trying to get on a tinny with three dogs and two cats was, nah, that's not going to happen.

My wife and I were feeding the neighbour's chooks and birds for a while.

We've also got a daughter with mild intellectual disability. I've got to consider that as well. Next time I might not be able to go down, but if I can, I will be there.

The water is rising now and one thing I've done is started posting information from the SES and the BOM so people have got accurate information coming in about what's going on; if they're well informed, then they can make a decision about what they can and have to do.

The problem with the 2022 floods is that most of the water came from Millfield and Laguna, from the south.

Our problem was, with no early warning system directly north of Broke, we had no idea what was coming. Plus the perfect storm part of it was out of Monkey Place Creek and Yellow Rock Creek. It was under a torrential rain and it flooded and Monkey Place Creek came up to the village before Wollongong Brook came over the road.

You couldn't do anything or go anywhere. I know a lot of people do worry, but at least they're happy with getting some information that's going to help them make a decision.

For me personally, it has been painful at times. For me, is what it is, that's how I look at it. You've just got to work on it, get over it, and move forward. You can sit back, like some people and say, 'I won't see it again in my lifetime,' but you just don't know.

In my immediate future I want to retire, but I will keep doing what I'm doing with regards to the community. We're busy this year with the Bicentennial stuff and then, I'll reassess what I'm doing with regards to the community. But I'll be involved somewhere.

After 200 years I think Broke is in a good spot. Even once the mines go, in about 30-or 40-years' time, it's going to be around because of the wineries and other tourist things starting to come. I think it's going to flourish. I really do.

Initially, down at the hall, there was no power. Once the power went back on, they started logging all the jobs and then it was 700 or 800 jobs that we did in the space of two weeks or 16 days. Everything from sewer pumps to washouts to getting air cons tested to make sure they work. If they don't work get them disconnected. It was an amazing amount of work and tradies that were around were fantastic. Absolutely phenomenal how much work people do.

I've got a folder with a heap of photos. One of our guys here put a drone up and on day two of the floods he took some drone footage. When you see a photo from the air, it gives you a good indication of how bad this was and how much it affected places. That's the one that I take out with everything about what happened in it.

From that experience, I learned that life is precious. You've got to live each day to the fullest and rely on your mates, especially when people have to rely on their mates to get through it.

After coming from where we used to live in suburbia, where it's very insular, you're living on your own block, in your own bubble, to come out here and have great mates and friends, and it is good to have that.

You've got to, you've got to have it.

Broke is home now. My wife and I talked about it, and I said, 'You're taking me out in a pine box feet first.'

What I know now is that family is important. Sometimes I need to be reminded, because I keep getting involved with other projects, but I always come back to that.

Family is important.

EVELYN HARDY

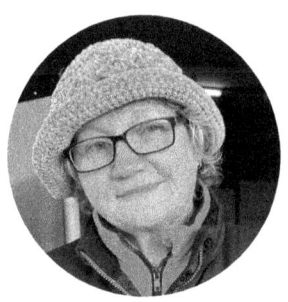

Evelyn's inspirational story is one of dedicated service to her community. As the secretary of the Broke Community Hall and a member of the Broke Residents Community Association, Evelyn was at the centre of the support during the flood in July 2022. Together with other community members and some service organisations, she helped provide various essential services, including communications, food, and loving support.

'Being there for the ones still going through this is very important to me personally, and providing support and wellbeing is a top priority moving forward,' says Evelyn.

Other community members recognised her tireless efforts as she put aside her needs after her house flooded and worked tirelessly for others. They call her a 'local legend.'

She is also involved in the recovery activities, which have been very difficult as many people, nearly two years later, are still not over the impact of the flood.

'It was very hit-and-miss as to where the worst or minor damage happened. I always say that minor and major damage causes the same mental damage to everybody.'

I've lived in Broke for 39 years. Both my kids were born and raised in the area. We had an everyday community life; kids went to school, playgroup and gardening. I worked until about 12 years ago when I had an accident at work. Once I got over that, I ended up at the Neighbourhood Centre. That was seven years ago this month.

Then, about four years ago, I had another accident that really hurt. The first accident took me six years to get back and move forward. But when the second accident happened, I was non-weight-bearing for four months and had to learn to walk again.

It took a toll, and I was knocked down mentally and didn't know whether I had the strength to get back up again. I realised I needed to focus on myself and getting my health and my mental health back. I reached out to people, so I didn't feel sorry for myself. I thought, I can't feel sorry for myself, so I refocused on who needed a hand. If I help them, it's going to help me as well. I began to help others see that they could move forward. We can't let accidents and things stand in our way.

I needed to get involved with the hall and get it to start breathing again, so I started up the morning cup of tea chat on the last Wednesday of every month to get people to come together. I could keep an eye on how the community felt and link them to different people and organisations, which I thought could help. That was cruising along, and then the BRCA (Broke Residents Community Association) was born, and I became involved.

I started putting things in place and pushing out there, interacting with people and finding out how they were, and it made me feel I had a purpose. It was hard going, and still to this day, especially when my leg gives me heck, and I wonder, can I keep doing this? Helping others helped me.

When the flood happened, that pushed things out.

The way I approached my self-healing, the whole community also had to do that. Many people were knocked down, and they are still being knocked down. It's a case of trying to pull them back up. There's not much

I can do to get their houses fixed, but I can certainly make sure that they are in a happier place where they can escape and don't have to think about all the cleaning up, and they will be cleaning up for quite a while.

Collectively, the flood knocked the whole community to its knees. It's gradually starting to pick up again.

I remember the first Christmas after the flood when we were all still in a big mess. The BRCA decided to put on a community Christmas. We called it 'Christmas with the Neighbours.'

Wow, what an event. It brought everybody together. Some people would not have Christmas like they used to, but it was incredible. A dear friend of mine and I—both our houses were wrecked—said, 'Let's put Christmas lunch on at the hall for the people who won't be doing Christmas'. So we did. We had sponsorship, and a local restaurant chef put on beautiful parts of the meal. Close to 40 people had Christmas lunch in the hall, which was lovely. We wanted to make things as normal as possible in a very much not normal situation.

Now, this was my flood experience. The 5th of July was like any other rainy day. We decided to go to town because there was nothing else to do. My son and I shopped, then thought we had better go home; it looked a bit wet.

We got to Broke and decided to go down to all the access roads into Broke and check how things were going. By that stage, the water had come up on the Wollombi road; that was nothing unusual; it was high, but it was okay.

We thought, yeah, it'll be fine. Then we went over the Milbrodale bridge, where it usually stabilises, checked everything, and returned. Then we drove around to make sure everybody was all right and went down to the common to see if anyone was camping and get them out or move them.

We were heading towards the fire shed when my daughter-in-law came to find me to get the keys and unlock the hall she said, 'Broke is being evacuated.' That was around about quarter past five.

I had to go home and get the keys. I grabbed my laptop, put a few things in a bag, and left. I ran into my husband and said, 'Get back to the house. Start putting things up.'

I went to the hall, turned on the heaters and the urn, and people started to turn up. At about twenty to six, I got an SES message to say, 'Evacuate Broke Now.' It was too late. Every road was flooded. People started to come in, and it wasn't too long after that the power and water went off.

We were all in the dark, but we had enough hot water in the urn to have warm Milo at midnight. Two homeless guys came into the hall, and they were a blessing. One helped me look after and entertain any children with the preschool stuff: pencils, books, Play-Doh, you name it. He entertained all of them and got warm drinks for people.

The other fellow had a bank of lights and a battery that he set up so that we could see and not trip over anyone. He set it up so that people could recharge their phones to 50 percent so that everybody got a fair amount of reception on their phone, which was great.

Then, the night became freezing cold. It was terrible. A lady came in who was very sick; she was going to be medevacked out by helicopter, but at midnight, it was cancelled because of the weather. Then I got a frantic phone call from a neighbour asking if someone could come and get them.

They were sitting on their kitchen table, and they thought they would be all right, but they weren't. There was water all through the house, so the fire brigade had to bring them to the hall.

That was a crazy night. I've never seen anything like it, and I've never heard the corrugated iron or Colorbond fences breaking and the tin ripping from the force of the water. Tanks and garbage bins floated by all night. The whole area stayed dry, but across the road, there was water all under the hall.

I used the water at the back steps to indicate how high the water came, and the next morning, as I watched it, I knew when it was starting to recede, which was around about nine o'clock. It dropped about three centimetres. It stayed that way for a while and then started to drop again.

It was all a case of having to watch this and take it as it came because it was all new. No one in that hall, nor anyone living in Broke, had ever experienced water in the village.

The last big flood inundated the village in 1949. Two further churches are over from the church and right over from the hall. A local resident, his house, and cattle yards are between those two churches. When the water breached the road into the village, it went around both churches and that house in the middle, but it didn't touch them. It filled up the paddock behind the churches, flooded the hall, and then the rest of the village.

The churches and that little house were an island. It was really weird. None of us knew what to expect, and houses you expected to have flooded for sure didn't. Then others did. Our house flooded, and my friend's house down the road didn't flood but had such serious pier damage that it's ruined. It was very hit-and-miss as to where the worst or minor damage happened.

I sent Claude back twice, then he came back and said, 'I've done all that.'

I said, 'Did you get the bottom shelf in the library?'

He said, 'No.'

I said, 'Quick, go back, and for goodness sake, don't put the dog in the crate.'

It was strange that it happened, and I didn't think we would be impacted. I remember walking around talking to everybody in the hall, and some people said, 'Oh, I don't know what to think.'

It still never prompted me to think that my house would be impacted.

But about 2 am, I heard from a neighbour, and it was flooded all right. It still didn't really sink in until the next morning when I waded knee-deep into the house into the yard. It was just above my ankle, and you wouldn't think that amount of water could cause so much damage, but it did.

It was devastating.

I thought there was no point in being obsessed with what I couldn't control. I could get upset and tear my hair out, but all of us were in the same boat. I just had to concentrate on making sure everyone was safe and doing what I had to do. Even when I did see, it didn't sink in. To this day, it's surreal. It happened to someone else. It couldn't possibly be me.

I remember I was talking to the fire captain, poor girl. She'd only become the fire captain that week when she was thrown into a baptism of water, not fire.

She said, 'Give me a fire any day; this flood business is just horrible.' And it goes on and on. And the smell, that's something you'll never forget, it's revolting. I didn't have time to think about our personal stuff, house, and belongings. I didn't ring our insurance company until three, maybe four days after the event because it didn't happen to me. It was a bit of denial.

I'm incredibly strong, probably too strong; people can be too strong. I've had to put up a wall because, at times, I've had to do things I didn't feel like doing.

I constantly had my phone stuck to my ear. If I wasn't dealing with insurance-related things, I was dealing with community issues and helping people. I didn't go to work for about five weeks. Even then, I had to distance myself from what was happening in Broke, my home, and everything so that I could concentrate on work.

My work involves helping people with problems, but I had to be careful because even though some of them knew what I was going through, I had to be mindful that my problems were not their problems. I had to keep it from them so that I could work with and deal with them, and respect for them was paramount. Whenever I had my work hat on, that's what I had to think about. I had to learn to compartmentalise. My entire life, including my family, Broke, commitments, work, and everything else, had its little hat.

When I walked into the house, I saw what a heck of a mess it was—absolutely everything. Then I found photos that were a mess, but my neighbour next door, who was clever, said, 'Don't move them, give them to me.' He sat on his mum's lounge room floor and took each photo off itself.

I didn't lose one of those photos, but months and months down the track, I had other photos stored in a box ready to go. I lost the lot. They were very special photos. You wouldn't think a photo is heart-breaking, but it is. They are photos of an event, and I don't think I can get copies of them. I don't even know how to find the people who took the photos to get copies. It's silly things like that, but it's not silly because it's personal.

Other people might not understand that. They'll say it's just things; they don't matter. They don't matter, I suppose, because lives weren't lost. Material things don't matter. But sometimes, those material things have a terrible habit of jumping up and smacking you when you least expect it.

But I've lost everything except things in the cupboards. Anything that was low down is gone, and I've got to start all over again. But we've got to get a house built before I can get any stuff.

My friend down the road, they're to start on her house in about three weeks. We're still in the DA stage but are finalising the last things. I've been assured that work will begin immediately once I sign on the dotted line.

Every single day is Groundhog Day. Nothing changes. Then, when something happens, you question it, and you go, nah, nah. Something's going to come up and change all this back to whatever else was happening before.

You cannot trust what is happening. As far as loss is concerned, we had a beautiful garden. We've had weddings and photo sessions and everything in our garden. Most of it is destroyed. We've had to take down trees and completely pull out gardens. A hundred percent. For the new house to be built, trees, shrubs have to be removed. I don't know how I'm going to cope with that. Oh, it's just a tree. Yes, it is just a tree and a garden, but we created that garden from nothing. That's yet another thing that's going to be taken away.

What I miss most is control and autonomy in my home and surroundings. I have no surroundings except boxes and mess. I'm a big cook, I love cooking. It's nothing for me to put on a big meal and invite people.

Yeah. I miss my home.

It was gut-wrenching watching the community. Grown men crying, and ladies. I was at my son's place, and I'd be out at half past five, walking across the road. You'd see people starting to come in, and they're covered in mud. They were wandering around like lost souls.

Then you'd see the anger boil up. We had some services and people who came on board, big businesses, and Centrelink in the hall. People had come in wondering what to do next. Where do we go from here? It may fall into place, but seeing people wandering around was hard, not knowing what to do.

We had many people start picking up those pieces and guiding people in the right direction, and then someone suddenly burst into tears or was angry and yelled. Those emotions were justified, but it was a real tennis match, and you didn't know which one to follow.

It was hard to see normally strong people belted around every moment of every day. You'd see people start picking up because they had got what they could on track. The army boys came in with bulk coal, and trucks of stuff were being moved out. When people started to see action, especially around their own personal space, it made them feel a bit better.

We are still trying to pick up the pieces almost two years later. That's very hard to take. It's tough to say.

What worked best on a community level was that we had each other. We tried to keep everybody in the loop as best we could; some people reached out for that. There were various levels of help. Some others wanted to help, but it worked. It worked where each helped the other. Some people didn't want so much help. Others needed help that couldn't be provided immediately. Everybody tried their hardest to help wherever they could. I think that community is essential for overall mental health.

The media were excellent. A couple of them were brilliant to this day. They still step up now and then.

Those journalists were great. They helped in many ways simply by spreading the word. There were a couple of local men who never stopped contacting us and who spread the word. If we needed anything, it was there.

There was, 'Oh no, I don't want to talk again. I really don't want to go through this again.' The same old questions sometimes became tiring, but that depended on what we'd already experienced that day.

Some didn't quite get us right, but that's the story. Never let the truth stand in the way of a good story.

Overall, it was a positive experience. Without them, it would have been well and truly not noticed.

A dear friend of our son lives in Cessnock. He contacted us only this year to ask a question.

I said, 'I'll get onto it as quickly as possible, but I'm still dealing with our house issue, and I'll probably forget, not for long. I promise.'

He said, 'Well, what's the matter with your house?'

I said, 'It got flooded in July 2022, the big flood in Broke.'

He said, 'Oh my God, I didn't know.'

Cessnock is 24 kilometres away. I couldn't believe it, but some people don't turn on the news. It's understandable. I don't watch TV.

I was asked what we learned from this. It's a multi-pronged question. Many people now realise that community and family really are one word. We are there for one another, and we live in each other's pockets. We don't have to be involved 100 per cent; just know that we'll put our hands up and help you.

We are there. It doesn't matter who you are or what has happened that life can throw at you. The lesson learnt is that we are not alone, we are one big community. That lesson can be very valuable to know. For some people, it's in their nature to sit back at home and be happy to watch the world go by. That's fine for them to know that if things get tough, all they need to do is put their hand up and yell out, people are there. You're not alone.

Then, there are those at the other end of the scale who put their hand up and never stopped. They kept going to the point where sometimes there were a few collapses—enough is enough, I can't go any further. Then, it was a case of eventually picking themselves up and dusting themselves off. I've got this, I just needed a moment. I'm fine.

At both ends of the scale, whether you're the one who likes your privacy and your home base or the one that puts their hand up and wants to be out there, we all have our mental health, self-awareness and well-being. We're all on the same level there; everyone is the same. But knowing that everyone can be there for you is such an important thing, and Broke has got that etched into it; it really is there.

You mightn't see someone for six months, but suddenly, there you are; how are you doing? It's very important to know that we have a community family.

It's got better since the flood. There was always help, concern, and mateship when someone needed a hand. Now it's entwined into us, it's made it even more noticeable.

One of the media people said to me, only a week or so after the flood. 'So what happened? Do you think you will move? Do you think you don't want to be here anymore?'

I couldn't believe it; I said, 'What? No, no way. This is my home. I'm staying. I'm not going anywhere. It's broke, but we can fix it.' I didn't know I said that until it went everywhere, all across the country.

I didn't mean to do that, but it's true, we are fixing it.

Broke has changed. It was always quite lovely, private, whatever you wanted it to be. It's grown. Look, places grow. Where you go doesn't matter. People move in and out, and business goes. But Broke has grown in a very positive way. It's owned by locals and non-locals, and everyone supports everybody else. If someone says, 'Oh, I'm, or we're doing this,' half the Broke people support it because it means a lot to support one another, whether it's a business or whatever, it's done in a positive way.

I want to see the hall keep growing. We're getting more and more bookings and especially when this refurbishment happens, it'll be a whole new facelift. We've got many, things happening. Broke's going to be the place to be in October. We started the year and then we had the Festival of Small Halls, which was a pretty amazing night.

We've got all these little things happening.

Broke is coming up to 200 years old and it's going to be one big Back to Broke party. There's lots of those kinds of plans, but I want to see the cup of tea, morning cuppa and chat still remain. I want to encourage small community events, bingo nights, all the little stuff that gets you together.

I want to encourage people to hire the hall. Have weddings, seminars. It doesn't matter what it is. I'd like to see life well and truly pumped into the hall, community wise, to become a base, a hub for the community and then there's all manner of things happening around the village.

Those who are old enough remember the dances that used to happen there. Over time that all fell off, it wasn't quite so community minded or based. What happened reawakened many memories, many things. Then of course, the different things we introduced to help the community has prompted people to become more focused again on what the hall can do for the community as a whole. It has reawakened the what the hall used to be and what the hall can be.

This flood will be remembered as the big one, it supersedes the '49 flood. Not too many people are still here who remember the '49 flood; their parents certainly would have been here, but there was a different layout of the village. There weren't fences, or roads in the way they are now, or as many houses, so the impact wasn't as dramatic.

This flood, however, took out houses, took out cars, washed out roads. It doesn't matter what direction you look. It was huge. Erosion ponds, houses with massive big holes under them.

This one will be remembered for simply that. When it came, it came big. Mr Watts, the old fellow that used to live in our house, was saying the water came up at sundown and the dog and I sat on the kitchen table till sunup.

And he just swept the mud out of the house and carried on. Well, the house is no more. It will have to be demolished.

It's a different dynamic as well. I think the 2022 July flood is going to go down in history and not be forgotten in a hurry.

What I would personally like to see, one, I'd like my house built. That'd be nice. I want to get my personal life, everything, all in place and all my ducks in a row.

In my new house—and I'll tell anyone this, I've said it to hundreds—no way on this earth will I ever have carpet in my house again. It's revolting. You get flood mud over a carpet, it's disgusting. So no carpet!

I want everything fixed. This hall is important; its refurbishment and facelift is about to start.

When all that's happened, I want to see Broke remain the very community-focused village it is. I'm sure that will happen because many of the people who live in the area live in the village, and they are the kind of people that want to see things go forward. They want to see positive stuff. They want to see growth and encourage people to come and enjoy our lifestyle. Then they can go home, know that was a really beautiful place to stay, they had a wonderful time. It hasn't impacted on us as the village that everyone loves, without it being impacted by big growth.

The best thing that happened for me is I have gained strong friendships. We're a group of ladies who would rock up to the hall, covered in mud, freezing cold, trying to feed people or whatever in their businesses, like B and B's, all manner of things.

We just gravitated towards one another. I didn't know any of them, personally. Now, we try very hard to catch up every month or every two months. We get together and we talk about it, we support one another, we help one another, we're there, we're sort of like our own group counsellors. Absolute undying friendship. Beautiful deep friendship. Those that helped, we helped each other.

The hall was the recovery centre. We developed friendships there, and contacts. Years ago, I could never initiate a conversation or be here talking like this. I wouldn't even pick up a phone. My self-esteem was low.

Now I might go, 'Oh, do I really have to, I'll be fine. I'll get in there.' I dust off and I'll keep going. I work because at the end of the day, I need to see results. If I can work towards doing that, that's the end game for me.

I see a job completed and I feel so good about the best results from that.

I'm pretty sure groups of people seeing a job well done or their personal jobs, whatever they're facing in their life, has got to be the grandest of feelings. That's got to be a plus, that the best thing to come out of all this is that people have moved on and are putting their best foot forward now.

Some people have a really healthy outlook. Others are still working towards that, but I have every faith that they can achieve their best moving forward place.

I must say the people around me are still very focused on the outcome of the health of Broke and are still the best people. They are an amazing bunch of people and very resilient. Mind you, we had a few crashes, like chucking willies and everything, but that's human nature.

If you want to cry, have a cry. We all know that we've got each other's backs and that's what's very important. They are a great bunch of people.

We could never do it individually. That would be a big load to carry. And that's why I think, like the girls when we reached enough, we unburden on each other and each other's problems, just let it out there.

If, as a group, people working together, shouldering the load, we get together and we can sort out different problems, it's the best way we can. If you did that on an individual basis, it couldn't be done. It's too much. We would individually crash and burn, but by sharing the load we're helping one another.

We do what we can for each other. I believe with that strength and keeping on showing people that strength, they can do it. You can do this. It's not going to be fixed in five minutes, moments down the track.

There's a little milestone coming up soon after an event. There is a wall coming up that's going to be hit and some people will climb the wall and other people will hit the wall. You drag them away from that and make them realise that what you're feeling is normal. You can move on.

We can do this and you'll be fine. Early days, but we'll be doing it. We can do it!

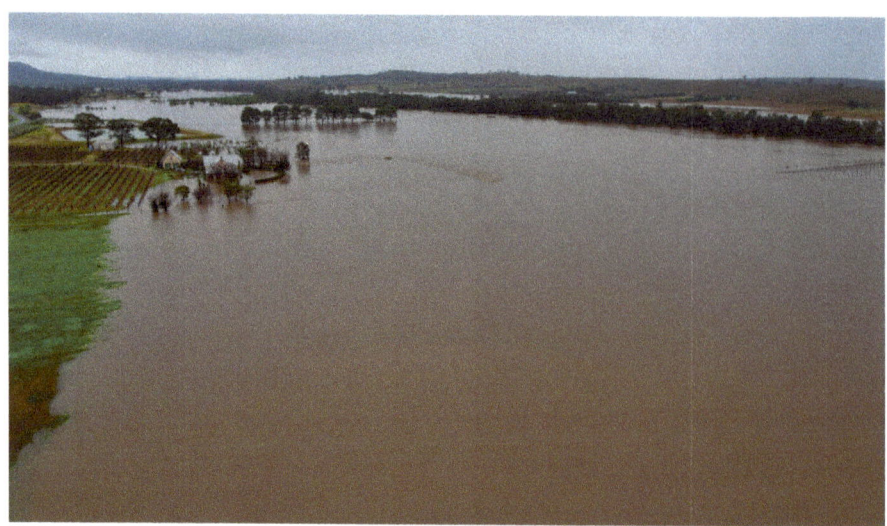

Vineyard properties between Milbrodale Rd and the Wollombi Brook. Most of the vineyard is underwater. Photo courtesy of Stewart Ewen

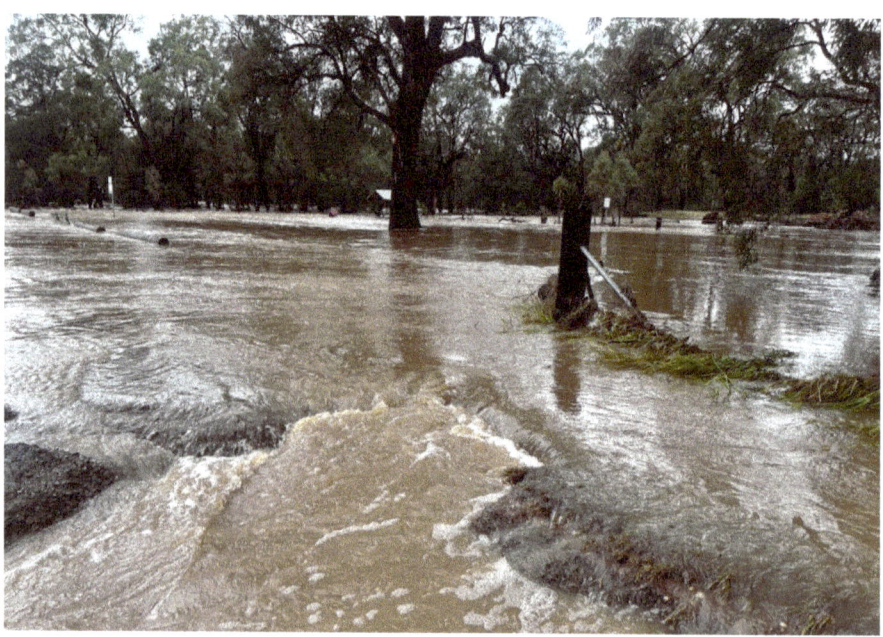

Water flowing over the Milbrodale Bridge showing the sealed road breaking up. Photo courtesy of Stewart Ewen

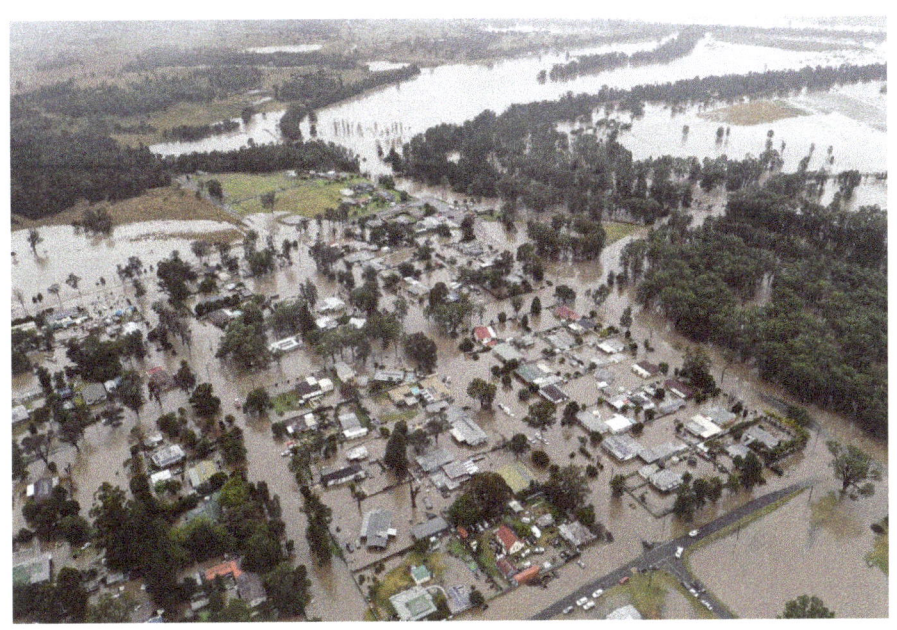

Aerial view of Broke. Photo courtesy of Stewart Ewen

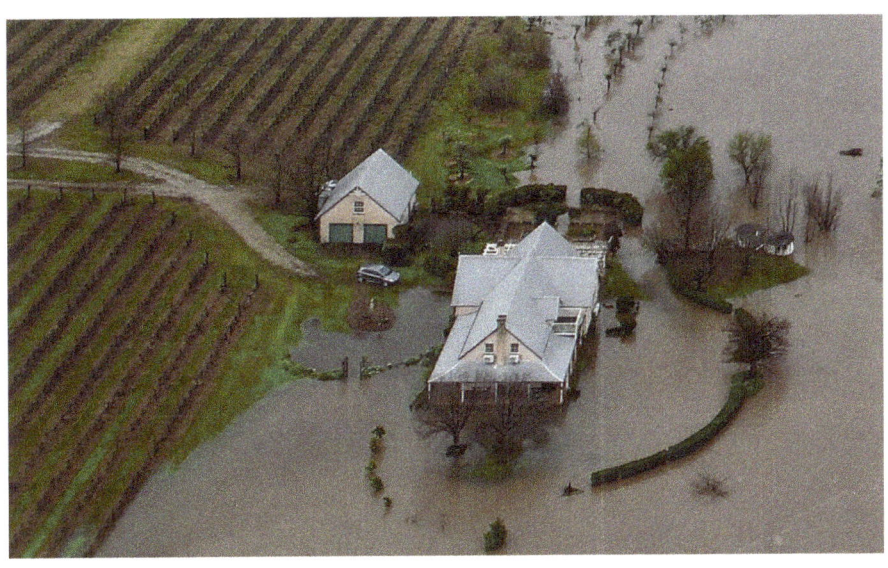

A Milbrodale Rd vineyard property. Water came within half a brick of flooding the house. Photo courtesy of Stewart Ewen

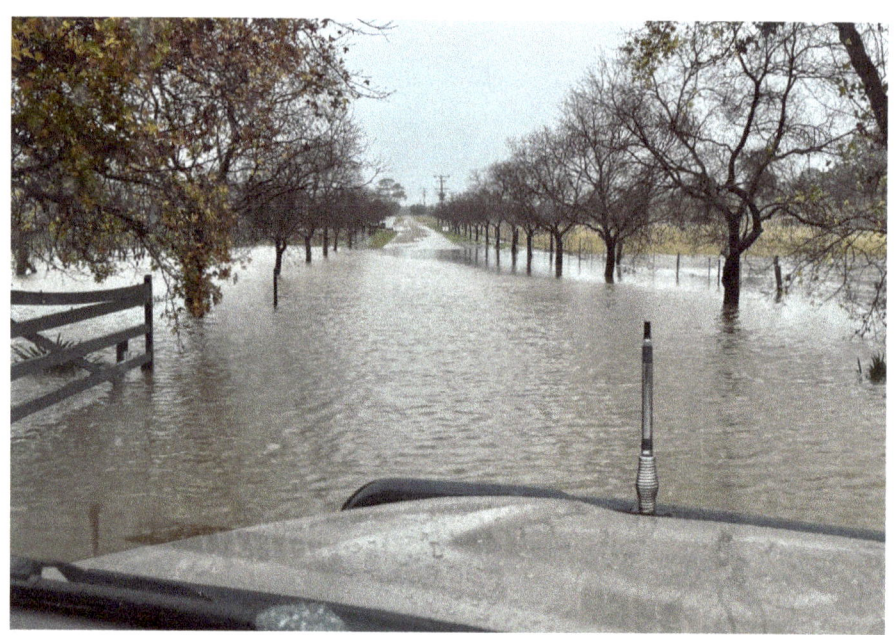
Milbrodale Rd outside Nightingale Vineyard. Photo courtesy of Stewart Ewen

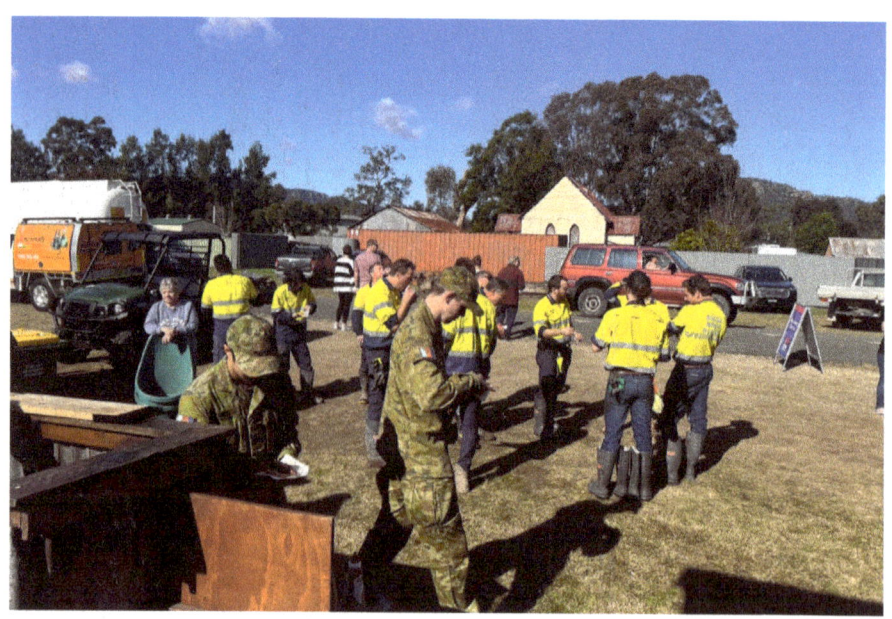
SES workers outside Broke Community Hall. Photo courtesy of Stewart Ewen

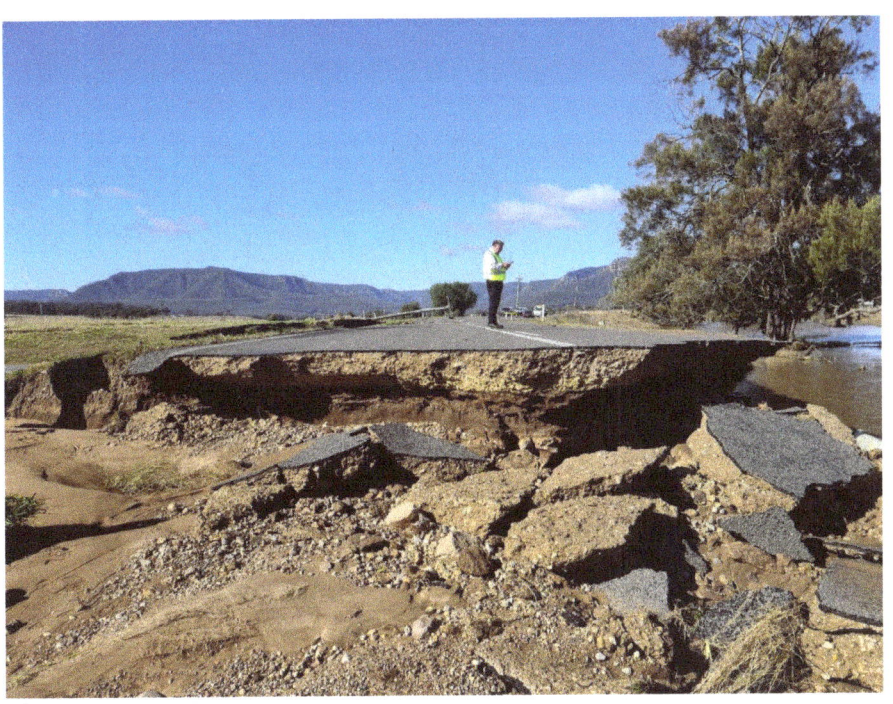

Broke Rd between Singleton and Broke. It took over 18 months to repair the road. Photo courtesy of Stewart Ewen

ANNIE COSSINS

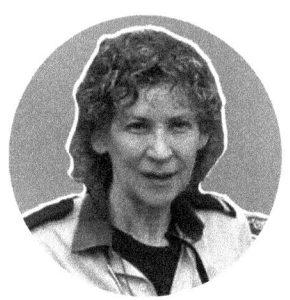

Annie is a volunteer firefighter and deputy captain with the Wollombi Brigade in the Lower Hunter District. During the floods in 2022, along with many other firefighters in the Wollombi Brigade, she undertook the daunting task of cleaning out local residents' flooded homes and businesses.

She learned how important it was for residents to start the recovery process amidst their tears, leftover fears and sense of hopelessness.

The floods didn't affect her home because she lives on a hill, although the sight of the tiny creek on her road turning into a river the width of the Hunter was something she hopes never to see again.

From both her personal perspective and role in the RFS, Annie's story captures the dedication, commitment, and compassion of the local volunteer organisations that are the bedrock of rural communities.

'Because we were surrounded, there was no way in or out. The SES couldn't get to us. The RFS Wollombi Brigade, became the flood clean-out group. We started calling ourselves the Rural Flood Service because we cleaned out about 40 structures: houses, sheds, and the pub.'

I've lived in Wollombi full-time for five years, although I've had a property here for 24 years. Part of owning a rural property is dealing with the two dangers for us: fire and flood. When I joined the RFS 12 years ago, I didn't imagine that part of our work would be flood work.

In 2022, my house wasn't affected at all. Things like roads and external infrastructure were affected, most of us were flooded. We couldn't drive out anywhere during the major flood on the 6th of July.

During that flood, the second-highest recorded level of the Wollombi Brook was 14.3 meters. Everything on the floodplain was affected.

Unfortunately, it affected the Wollombi pub, which is an iconic part of our village, as well as all the houses alongside the Brook. People love building there because it's picturesque, but they went under.

Because we were surrounded, there was no way in or out. The SES couldn't get to us.

The RFS Wollombi Brigade, became the flood clean-out group. We started calling ourselves the Rural Flood Service because we ended up cleaning out about 40 structures: houses, sheds,

and the pub.

It's very confronting work. When floodwaters enter a house, the violence and power of the water tips everything on its head. I can remember walking into places where all the couches, refrigerators, and everything else had been tossed into the middle of the room.

Floods enter at full volume, and when they leave, everything drops. Flood victims always talk about the inches—not millimetres— the inches of mud left behind, which contains all sorts of bacteria.

Our job was to remove all the furniture, the sodden carpets, everything we could. We spent hours and hours hosing out the mud, so it was physically tough work. We had a lot of help from the Defence Force in Wollombi, from young men stationed at Singleton, most of whom had only recently joined the Defence Forces. They were great to work with, very willing and capable. We ended up being a great team together.

When we train, we train to be bushfire firefighters. That's our job. Then we can do further training to become village firefighters, we do many things: bushfires, structure fires, vehicle fires, any vehicular accidents we come across. Quite a lot of vehicles crash around here, mostly tourists.

In 2019, we had the biggest fire campaign around Wollombi in our history because, at one stage, we were surrounded by four fires.

We've only recently started to engage in flood rescue work. The RFS has sent each brigade a series of flood rescue kits. We're not like the SES; we won't necessarily be trained to do swift water rescue. That's on the cards, but at the moment, we have the equipment and capacity to do rescues while we're on land and someone is trapped in water. Some brigades will be issued with a flood boat.

We'd really like a flood boat, and I'm not sure if we might be getting one. That would assist us in this community, in events like the East Coast low we had the other day. Who would have thought? We were not nearly as badly affected as the Illawarra, Wollongong, and some places in Sydney, but this is the problem. We don't know when the next East Coast low will come. They are certainly much more frequent during autumn and winter. A flood boat would be great for our and the community's safety. We'll have to wait and see whether we get one.

The floods impact people in the community in different ways. For example, I know the people who live on Paynes Crossing Road, which leads to Broke. They were impacted for a very long time because they're often flooded in for around three weeks.

I've got friends who live in Bucketty, a little area south of Wollombi. Their electricity had been cut off. They had a generator, but they'd run out of fuel. It's hard living when you've got no electricity or lighting. You can't access water because we are all on tank water, so we depend on electrical pumps to pump water from our tanks into our kitchens and bathrooms.

I'm lucky, I've got my own storage capacity, so I don't lose electricity if the general infrastructure goes down.

Life can get basic when you don't have electricity and can't access water. Then, people can't be contacted because phone lines are down, and they can't charge their mobile phones. Things do get a bit compounded.

I think after that experience, people have rethought what they need to do for the future. Maybe getting a better generator, stocking up on fuel, or getting battery power so they've got power when the grid goes down.

Our clean up work was very challenging, but I'm an experienced firefighter and deputy captain. It's not a job you learn to switch off. I also used to do very confronting work in my day job, so I just got on with the job.

We're trained to get on with the job, but I retain the capacity to see a homeowner's distress. Not everyone does that, it depends on who you are. I'm happy to give people a hug if that's what they need. I had a homeowner who was in tears all the days we were at her house.

That's fine for me. I'm not confronted by people's pain or their emotions. It's part of the job. You do what you can. We always consulted with people. 'What do you want us to do? What do you want us to save?' We're very respectful because the disaster of a flooded house is confronting. It's shocking because we all go back to our houses and think, my God, that could have happened to us.

It's the same with fires. My experience in the RFS is that the people I work with are efficient and get on with the job. We know what to do, we're compassionate, and we know we are there for the right reasons because if we weren't there, who was going to do it?

When someone is faced with a flooded house, if they can't get rid of the mud, they have no starting point. There are inches of mud. Sometimes, it goes right up to the walls. I can remember walking into a bathroom where everything was caked in mud. They don't have the correct hoses, pumps and power that we have to get rid of the mud. Getting everything out that's been destroyed, like couches, TVs and refrigerators, is a big help for them because moving big fridges and couches is tough on your own or for two people.

We've got many strong people who can do that and then get rid of the mud, so they can

decide what to do and whether they have to re-gyprock the house. It also allows everything to dry out. Maybe they can go to a neighbour or live upstairs until the downstairs dries out. We can pull out the kitchen, or whatever they want so they can start from scratch.

Everyone was grateful we were helping. There were tears, but everyone was grateful that we

were there. I don't mind the physically demanding and confronting work. It's what I signed up for.

As far as I know, governments don't employ staff to come and sort out flooded houses or structures. The RFS and the SES are important services. It would cost the state government millions of dollars to employ the number of people who volunteer for them.

We feel a sense of achievement. Perhaps there is a human need to help others. We get the sense that it's a disaster for that particular family, but we've helped them take the first step to recovery.

Many people don't know what to do; they don't know where to start because they're so emotionally impacted. They're fretting and anxious and still recovering from the trauma of perhaps being in the house when it was flooded and wondering if they were going to survive.

They're dealing with a lot of traumas. We can come in and help, not so much help them with the trauma because we're not psychologists. What we can do is help restore, to some extent, normality, or take the first steps towards normality. That allows them psychologically to see that there is a pathway out of the trauma. That's the way I see it, anyway.

If a homeowner could, they would work alongside us and then come back the next day, and we could see how much we'd already done and how much more they might've done overnight.

Then, they would have other chores for us to deal with. It can take a year or more for people to get back to their situation before the flood. But it's creating that pathway for them, and then they can get in the builders, carpenters, kitchen designers, or whoever to fix the place up. Maybe redo the flooring, put in a new kitchen, and so on.

I know one couple who had to move their house, and they've managed to do that. Their recovery has been a two-year process, but if they didn't move the house, it would end up being flooded again at some point. It can be a very expensive process because most people we helped out weren't insured because they're on the flood plain.

I don't know if people get used to the trauma of their situation. I know some people have been flooded time and again, and they still live where they are. I expect they might be used to what will happen up to a certain point. It's still traumatic, though.

I know one family who didn't want our help. They'd been flooded several times before and knew exactly how to clean up. They had children and a large extended family to help them out, so they were prepared to do it to live where they lived.

The advice I would offer people regarding preparation depends upon where they live. If they live around Wollombi, they're on the floodplain. Some people still live in the flooded houses, so they know they're vulnerable again.

The best thing would be for them not to continue to live on the floodplain. They must leave for their safety before another flood happens. Certainly, for people whose houses weren't affected but were flooded in, they need to have the equipment, which is a monetary outlay.

I had to spend a lot of money on storage batteries. I recommend, and most of us do this anyway, having the sort of food in your pantry that allows you to eat for three weeks. If the electricity goes, everything in the fridge and the freezer will eventually not be edible.

You need lots of fuel if you're dependent on generators. Some people use their generators for a few hours each day to keep the fridges running, and then overnight, the fridge is cold enough to keep their food.

Some people can't afford to move, that's one of our problems too. Unless there's a government buyback scheme, some people will experience floods in the future.

What can a community do? Around our community at the moment, there is funding to create a network of UHF radios so that people can still communicate if their landlines die and they can't charge their mobile phones.

That's a good outcome around here. I don't know how many people are involved in it, but if other communities try to think about it, how can they help each other? How can they find out if the elderly ladies or gentlemen who live on their own are going to be okay?

That's certainly a great initiative. I know it was government money, and it was called the MEPCC scheme, but that's all I know because I haven't been involved in administering it. But the network works and people do check up on each other.

They all have a time to call in once a week. It can be used throughout the year, for example, for medical emergencies or any emergency, not fire and flood.

Many things could be done to improve the area impacted by the floods. If there was an unlimited budget, I'd certainly think about the state of the roads because one of the big issues for isolated valleys that were flooded was that they lost their roads. We don't have bitumen roads. The main road through to Cessnock is bitumen, but most of us live on gravel roads, which are an absolute disaster to negotiate during floods.

Some people have their whole roads washed away, which is terribly dangerous. They have to fork out for that expense unless it's a council road. I'm lucky; I live on a dirt road, but it's a council road, so they repaired it.

I'd love to see my road become a bitumen, and other roads too. They also get ruined but are usually more passable than a gravel road.

I'd have many more people and rescue boats out here. If we'd had boats and people trained to deal with those boats in floodwaters, we could have helped many more people sooner, with access to food and medication, things like that.

I'd offer the money to buy back the houses of people on the floodplain if that's what keeps them there so that they could move elsewhere if they choose to. Living there and constantly worrying about the next flood is not good for people and makes them much more vulnerable.

Some of the crossings over our creeks. I get flooded in because where my road crosses the creek, it's a causeway, not a bridge.

We can do much more by repairing bridges and ensuring they are high enough to prevent flooding. Many bridges around here were flooded. I don't know how high is high enough, but it would certainly be better than what we've got at the moment.

We could give everyone who lives in the area a UHF radio for free. We could provide more money to the RFS and the SES for their equipment for dealing with floods. We've only got the basics at the moment, which is good, but I'm sure we could get more sophisticated stuff.

You'll often hear politicians say, we're a very resilient community. People naturally are resilient wherever they go, and that resilience will vary from person to person, household to household, but everyone wants to pick up the pieces and return to their normal lives.

It seems to be a natural human instinct. I see it over and over again. There is naturally a period where people fall apart emotionally, but then they gradually get it together and start rebuilding in whatever small way they can. That's what humans do.

If there's someone to help another person along the way, isn't that what we do as humans? That's the whole point of having voluntary organisations. Why do people volunteer hours and hours and hours of their time for free?

It has to be this human instinct to assist, to help. If you help others, you're also helping your community. The thing that you're fundamentally a part of.

What inspired me most during the flood was the teamwork between the RFS and the army chaps. They were very willing and incredibly respectful, particularly as I was a woman in charge at the time. The community's willingness was inspirational.

Many people came out and helped the former pub owners clean out the pub to try and get that back up and running. There was probably less community engagement with their neighbours, but that might've been because they thought we would end up doing the job.

We could do that because of our equipment. When disasters happen, people are very good at working as a team and not worrying about their egos.

I was only disappointed by a couple of homeowners in one place, but I wouldn't worry about that too much. That was the most challenging place we dealt with. I won't say too much about that. No matter what happens, there will always be difficult people, whether you go shopping in Woolies or in a major disaster.

It's important to be able to put that aside and keep doing what you're doing because humans are great, but they can also be difficult. You've got to be able to deal with both the good and the bad and not let that affect your work. I do what I do, then I go home, talk to the cats, and watch telly or something. You've got to find a way to come down from that.

The RFS has a phone line with people who are there 24 hours a day if we've attended a critical incident, so that support is there. I usually talk to friends and other firefighters. It's always good. Sometimes black humour gets you through. You've got to be able to laugh during a crisis to help you keep going.

One of the advantages, of course, is having a peaceful place to come home to without any crazy stuff around. That's what helps me. You've always got to talk to someone who's on the same wavelength as you, someone who's got enough empathy to hear what your particular trauma or sadness is.

There's certainly enough of them around for me. There are many local groups in Wollombi that do different things, and I'm a part of a couple of others. I help out with some of them if they need it. There's a lovely community here. I'm part of a terrific group of women, and they're nice, easy-going, and fun people. It's lovely and it's something you don't get in the city. You can live in the street for a couple of decades and still say hello to the neighbours but not engage more than that.

Here in Wollombi, everyone stops for a chat. It's a very different state of mind. People want to connect in a village, and it's lovely.

The long-term future of the community is an interesting question because many of us are in our senior years. Many landholders around here are in their 60s and over. One day, we're not going to be around. Unfortunately, land prices around here escalated during COVID, so it's tough for younger people to move in unless they inherit their parent's property. Younger people can't buy in with an ordinary income.

It's a great community to live in, but it's limited in that we have to travel a long way to go to a doctor, let alone a hospital. There are always limitations to living in rural areas. You have to love it out here to accept those limitations.

What will happen when many landowners here will either be in nursing homes or possibly in the grave in the next 20 years? I think about that myself. Given that these properties are not particularly cheap, I don't know who will buy them. We discuss this question, but we don't have any answers.

There is also the question of who's going to run the RFS, SES, and local organisations. We need younger people to join. The occasional younger person does join, but we need more.

I definitely enjoy being in the RFS. I enjoy the camaraderie, teamwork, and connections with other people, and there are a lot of interesting things you can do there.

I do more than firefighting; I'm also involved in several other ways. Some people are happy to turn up to the odd fire call, while others get more involved; it's up to the individual.

The best thing about being here is the peace and quiet. After living in Sydney for nearly 40 years, I find the noise of Sydney unbelievable. It is an underlying stress that never goes away. Whereas I'm looking out my door now, I've got incredible views. It's all green. It's incredibly quiet. It's paradise out here.

If people have anxiety or stress problems, come to the country because it all dissolves away. Life is much more about the weather, the environment, and the associated difficulties. Still, it's also much more rewarding than living in a city. That's my view anyway. I know some city folk wouldn't be able to cope with that, though.

The Wollombi Brigade is a great brigade. We are very engaged with the community. We've had a philosophy for many years of holding workshops to educate people about what to expect. To have a plan, create a safe environment around their house, make their house safer and when to leave if that's what they choose to do and the dangers of staying.

Of course, deep inside, I fear losing my home because I've seen houses lost. Everyone around here has that fear in the back of their minds, yet we still live here, so we are willing to take the risk.

I often tell friends and neighbours, 'Your house is vulnerable. You could do X, Y, Z to make it less vulnerable.' In our area, we only have eight fire trucks, and there are 300 to 400 properties out here. It's easy to do the maths. We will be there when we can.

One of my cats was very traumatised during the 2019 fires because my house was under threat. My whole property was burnt, except my house. In a way, I've been there and done that, but I am also aware that it could happen again. It's not that you become blasé; you become prepared. Each year, I do more and more to improve this property to make it bushfire-safe. It's already flood-safe, but that's what people have to do.

Some ignore the risk, but the best thing is to be prepared. And if the worst happens, it happens, but that's all we can do as humans anywhere. It's so much better talked about; it's better to have it out in the open.

We're always happy to visit people's places and advise them on how safe their property is. People should consult with the RFS more and ask them to come and look at their houses. People often store a lot of stuff under the house, like timber, old building materials, firewood, etc.

We can say a lot about how to make a house safer, but there's no guarantee. It can be very difficult if the flood washes out a lot of stuff from under a house; it is a hazard for anyone coming in to help clean up.

The members of the RFS are here to help and support the community.

CHRIS BOOKS

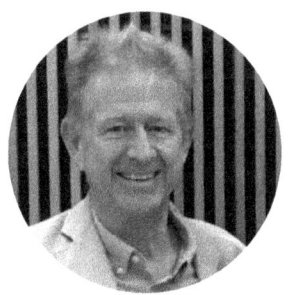

Chris Books, who was the owner and proprietor of the iconic Wollombi Tavern during the July 2022 flood, is a resilient and community-oriented individual. In the early eighties, when he was in the army he discovered the tavern during regular trips to Singleton.

In 2016 he and his wife decided to buy a small hobby farm around two hours from Sydney, then found the property they liked in Wollombi. 'I said to my wife, "I want to buy my little piece of Australia." We lived in this stupid big house in Sydney, but we knew only the two people next door to us and people across the road.'

In 2017 and passionate about preserving local history and traditions, Chris took on the challenge of running the historical pub. His commitment to Wollombi and its residents reflects his deep connection to the area and his unwavering dedication to preserving its unique character.

Wollombi is a small village, 'two hours from Sydney, but a long way from anywhere'. The tavern is one of the major focal points for the local community. For tourists, it's the biggest attraction in the village.

Despite facing numerous adversities, including bushfires, floods, and COVID lockdowns, Chris remained dedicated to the tavern and the community it served. As a volunteer firefighter, he embodies the spirit of service and resilience, facing challenges with determination and positivity.

After buying our property in Wollombi, we gradually became weekenders. We used to come up on Friday night and go back down on Sunday afternoon. Then, when I bought the pub, we extended that to Mondays. After about a year of owning the pub, my wife said, 'Why don't we just move up there permanently?' So, we did.

We sold the farm and bought a house in town, although town is a very loose word in Wollombi. It's a very small village, we're still on about five and a half acres here. We love the country lifestyle. We've both got elderly parents still alive, and a son who lives in Sydney, but we hate going to Sydney now.

It's been fun. Up here, everyone knows you, and you know everyone. As my wife said, 'If they don't know something about you, they make it up,' but that's fine. Communities like that pull together in these sorts of times.

No matter where I go, if somehow it comes up in conversation that I used to own the Wollombi Tavern, everyone would straightaway go, 'Oh, Doctor Jurd's Jungle Juice.'

We had a pretty rough trot of it because we had the bushfires of 2019 and 2020. We went from that into a flood in 2020. There was a flood that broke the bushfires, then we went into a first lockdown for COVID, came back out of that, and then went into the second COVID lockdown. We had a flood in March 2022 and the big flood in July 2022, where it came up to the top of the doors at the pub.

I'm just one of those people who doesn't get upset by things I can't control. I keep carrying on. I'm lucky to be a builder with another business in Sydney. Although I lived up here in Wollombi by then, I wasn't reliant on Wollombi for personal income. I had twelve staff who needed to be paid and looked after, so I looked after them and paid them even while we were shut. We were only closed for two weeks after the flood, then managed to reopen in a very wish-washy way, but we were open.

During the fires, the pub was the focal point. We set up the RFS community engagement at the pub so everyone could get into town and see what was happening the next day. Then, in the floods, everyone came down and helped us clean the pub out and get it open again.

To be honest, the flood in March 2022 probably made us a bit lackadaisical. The last big flood up here before 2022 was in 2007. Most people remember that weekend when the Pasha Bulker ran aground at Newcastle. In that flood, the water came up to about bar level.

In the March 2022 flood, the water came up to about a metre below the floor, but all our air conditioning units and a lot of our refrigeration are under the floor. We lost our refrigeration machinery. There was a fair bit of fixing up after that one, but it wasn't massive and didn't destroy us. We reopened within a few days.

When the July flood came, one of my staff members, who lives further up the creek and has lived here all his life, understood exactly what was happening. He rang me and said, 'This is going to be a big one.'

That was a couple of days before the flood because it took a while for the water to come down. The thing about floods is that they're insidious. They come very slowly. At least you can fight a fire. You can't fight a flood.

Because he told me it would be a big one, we put everything above bar level. We thought, if it's going to be bad, it can't be worse than 2007. Well, like I said, it was about a metre and a half higher than that and was the biggest flood since 1949.

Across the road from the pub is the museum, which is the old courthouse. It's got a brass plaque on the wall showing where the height of 1949 came to, which was probably about a metre below the July flood.

I knew the history of flooding in the town, but not as much as I know now. Some locals, born and bred here, tell you that it's flooded every year.

There's a saying in town, 'We actually like a small flood because small floods give us a bit of downtime, a bit of quiet time.'

You become a little bit blasé about them. Everyone who lives in this area has about a week's worth of food all the time because we know that it will happen every now and then.

This one was very different. I live a kilometre from the pub and would have had to put a boat in the water three times to get to it. Put it in, get it out, put it in, get it out.

When I first bought up here many years ago, I was told about how it floods. At one point, they proposed building a dam here and damming the valley. They only build dams where there's a lot of water.

You've got to be prepared. My house is high and dry, as are most houses in town. The lowest building in town is the pub. It's on about eight acres, but it's on a floodplain, so you can't do anything with it. But to give people an idea, if anyone ever goes up there and sees how low the creek normally is when it's running, the flood came through at over 12 metres, which is pretty high.

The other amazing thing is that everything floats away. Water tanks float away even if they're full of water, and outdoor furniture all floated away even though it's so heavy you can barely lift it. The ice machine floated, and the ice box floated away even though it was full of ice. And some gas tanks.

We don't have any services. We're on tank water, bottled gas, and septic. That's the horrible bit—a lot of septic tanks go under, and so the flood water is quite toxic. Then you have to clean out everything. There is a lot of work, but you just have to get on with it.

During the March flood, we sat at the back of the pub and drank some beer, watching the water rise. You don't ever expect it to get as high as it did. The peak of that flood was between midnight and one in the morning. I have a photo taken by the only local who could take a photo. He happened to take it at 12:30 am that day, so I've got a picture of the flood at its peak.

You look at it and stand there where the picture was taken. Look at it now, and people cannot believe it. It's a phenomenal amount of water in a very short time. In fact, we just had another flood last week. It was only a small one; it broke the banks, but not by much.

I suppose you get used to it. It's part and parcel of living here. Wollombi is an Aboriginal word for meeting of the waters because Wollombi Brook, which is the actual creek, has a north arm and a south arm, and they meet just north of Wollombi. Then it heads all the way up through to Broke and then all the way through to the Hunter River. It's a system that everyone understands.

If the Hunter River is flooding, the water coming out of Wollombi Brook has nowhere to go. It gradually backs up through Broke, back to us, and then back through Laguna. Then it's contained here because we're a very narrow valley with high hills on both sides and quite steep.

When it rains, it also depends on which way the rain comes. The little flood we had last week came from the northern brook, which is a bit different from the southern brook, where the pub is. It depends on which brook comes down as to who gets flooded and who doesn't.

I sound like a really well-versed local. I've been here for eight years now, and running the pub, I got to talk to many people, so I've become a bit of an expert overnight. It is just interesting. I'm in the local RFS, so I was also there for the bushfires.

If you couldn't put up with it, you would have to leave because you can't stop it. That's really the answer.

We had a guy here who settled on his property on the Friday before the flood, and it was one of the only houses that went under. After the March flood, the previous owner had paid a fortune to have floodproof doors put in on the lower level.

In July, the new owners bought it on the premise that it had floodproof doors, but they weren't floodproof.

As a builder, I can't imagine how you could build a workable hinge door that is floodproof. To make things waterproof, you must look at what's on board ships to make a weatherproof door.

The pub is a meeting place, and there's a core group of people who go to the pub regularly, and I know all those people intimately. Down at the next village, Laguna, which is only seven kilometres from here, is a wine bar. It's not actually a pub.

Many people go there. There are two groups of people, and there is a bit of cross-matching between them. In Wollombi is a T-intersection. You either go north to Broke and Singleton or south to Laguna and Sydney. Or east to Cessnock, and you can't go anywhere else. The pub sits right at the end of that intersection, so it really is the dead centre of town.

The pub is the driver of the town's economy because it's the only thing that attracts people; there are a couple of little cafes and other things, but it does drive the town. We are a tourist town. It's also a big cattle farming area around here. The town itself and the businesses rely on the fact that the pub is a big drawcard.

Everyone knows what the pub is and where it is—you can't miss it. It's not a very big place, but it used to be very big. Back in the 1950s, Mel Jurd, the famous Doctor Jurd, even though he was never a doctor, accidentally burnt the place down when he put petrol in the kerosene fridge. The story is that the community rebuilt the pub in six weeks.

That's how important it was to this area. I mean, it hasn't always been the only pub in the area; Wollombi had four pubs at one stage.

It was meant to be a big place until coal was discovered at Cessnock in Newcastle. That's when Wollombi got cut off. It was on the Great North Road.

Wollombi also had significance to the First Nations. I am told that Mount Yengo, just over the back of us, is Australia's second most sacred site, and there are many Aboriginal carvings around here.

But Wollombi is interesting because it doesn't belong to any one nation. That's why it was a meeting place. We have a little Aboriginal cultural centre in the middle of town, and they take people on tours.

When I arrived, I was determined not to change anything straight away but to take on board the place's history. It's not only the pub's history but the history of the town. The family I bought it from had been here since the 1800s.

I researched what I could about the pub back to the day they first built it. It was called Hawkesbury Hotel. It went through a few different incarnations before the current one, a two-story timber place. The original pub was sandstone and moved up here from around the Wiseman's Ferry, St. Albans area.

Wollombi is a quiet little town now, but it's been a boom-and-bust place as different industries came and went. At one stage, there was a massive dairy industry. There's not a dairy to be seen around here at all now. It was very much a logging industry place. One of the significant histories of the tavern itself was that land at the back. It was mainly used for the old bullocky guys coming up to pick up the timber. They camped overnight there and kept their bullocks at the back there, and then now it has done a bit of a turn back around to cattle; it's now beef cattle in small herds.

The main negative about the place now is that it's getting very expensive to live here, which is keeping the younger generation from being able to buy property. Our population of lawyers and accountants is bigger than anywhere else in Australia, all with holiday homes.

The other killer is these Airbnbs, and what have you. We have many of them now. People come up here and fall in love with the beauty of the place. It's a beautiful place and a quintessential cute little town.

After the flood, the streets were blocked, so the whole street, out the front of the pub, was a mass of people washing things, cleaning things, and working out what we would throw away. One of the biggest couple of things people don't even realise. I didn't realise either, to be honest, but everything that's used for food preparation had to be thrown away. Anything that cannot be successfully washed has to be thrown away. You lose things; you lose TVs, computers, printers.

But one of the worst things I never even thought of was that in the kitchen, we have deep-fat fryers. Because it's a pub, it does chips. All the oil comes out of the fryer and coats everything in this layer of oil, which is disgusting. It was slippery in there because kitchen floors are prone to being slippery anyway. The building wasn't damp, but we lost all the electrical goods.

The main reason it took us two weeks to reopen was that we had to redo all the electrics. But the building itself survived remarkably intact. Some doors swelled, but the building itself was good. The bar collapsed, but the beauty of that is that the people buying the pub off me would renovate anyway. In some ways, it saved money because a lot of stuff they were going to throw away was thrown away.

The council was excellent. They provided giant skip bins for us to put all the stuff in and remove it. My wife had rung the council to ask if they were sending someone out, and they said no. The next thing, Melissa, who works there, rang her back and said, 'I'll arrange for skip bins to come out, and you tell me when they're full, and I'll arrange for them to be picked up.'

We had to put everything in. I had locals come down with bobcats to help move the heavy equipment and put things in. We had to throw out fridges and stuff and the ice machine. We've lost three of them since we've owned the pub. In fact, the ice people said, 'We're not going to give you another one.' But I ended up talking them into giving me another. One of the iceboxes has never been found; it's big, and it holds 300 bags of ice.

The RFS wash out sheds and outbuildings, things that go under and still stay there, or they wash down tennis courts. A huge amount of detritus is left on tennis courts, and there's another thing that people don't see. There is a mob that will come out and pick all that rubbish off the fence for you, and they're volunteers.

The other big shout-out I've got to give to is the army. When the army turned up, it was so good to have these young blokes. They had just finished their recruit course and were up at Singleton waiting to be deployed to their regiments or wherever they were going to go. They had a young lieutenant and a couple of corporals, and they would do anything, even down to the lieutenant. Being ex-army, when he came up and said, 'What do you want me to do?' I said, 'Well, I won't ask you to do anything.' He said, 'No, I'm here to work too.' The army would do anything.

I don't know if people know what a pelican is. It is one of those white plastic cubes you see with the metal frame that carries water. One of them was on the roof of the pub.

An army boy said, 'What else do you want us to do?' I said, 'If you can get that down off the roof down for me, that'd be great.' I'm in my sixties now. Climbing on roofs is not for me anymore. Nothing was a problem for them. In fact, one of the ice boxes had floated away and tipped over on its back, so they climbed in to get all the ice bags out.

The goodwill of many people is fantastic. The first thing that happens here in a flood is when the fire brigade comes and hoses everyone's property. You've got to get rid of that mud. The mud is the killer; it stinks, and it sticks. You don't want to let the mud dry out. You've got to get into it while it's wet. As I said, being part of the RFS, I even left the pub for a few days and went and did my bit, hosing out other people's places.

We run the RFS on volunteers, but it is very demanding, and unfortunately for us up here, it's very much an aging membership of our RFS, and we are in a challenging area to fight fires because it's very steep and other fire brigades hate coming out to help us when we have a fire because no one realises just how steep it is here and we have no water.

With not having a supply of younger people living in the area, we're not getting the new people to replace the people we lose.

The RFS, like all organisations, is becoming more digital, which is scaring away older people. For instance, here at Wollombi, you no longer have phone connections when you drive within a kilometre in either direction from the pub.

We've got one Telstra tower in town, but even if you're a Telstra customer, you don't get reception. Heading to Sydney, you'll have to drive about 30 to 40 km before you have a mobile phone connection again.

People up here don't necessarily have smartphones. Even the government radio network, which is what the RFS, police, and ambulance all work on, doesn't work in half the valleys around here. The RFS were forbidden to go into certain areas during the fire because they weren't safe and because we had no communication. The people who lived in those areas weren't particularly happy.

That was not the case so much during the floods. You've still got the issue of no mobile phones, and they've stopped servicing landlines around here now, so people are dropped. I just dropped my landline because I don't need it anymore. The best thing that's happened here in a long time is Starlink. I don't want to give them a plug, but Starlink works and keeps going. We are on satellite TV here; we can't get TV reception. It's two hours from Sydney and a million miles from nowhere.

The biggest benefit of the flood is it reinforces the community spirit. We all know each other, and we need to help each other on a regular basis.

We've had elderly people around here—unfortunately, they've died now, but people used to go around and light their fire for them and make sure that they got out of bed okay that morning. You wouldn't see it in the city.

That's what it does. It reinforces that we are reliant on each other.

We look out for each other a lot and try to help each other as much as possible. I'm not saying everyone loves everyone around here—that's just impossible—but there are many good people here and everywhere in the world.

I lived in Sydney for 56 years, and during my childhood in the sixties, we used to go out until the lights came on. But nowadays, you don't even know who your neighbours are, let alone talk to them. I think that's the difference, and that's reinforced by natural disasters. Unfortunately, Wollombi is massively prone to flooding and equally massively prone to bushfires.

It's a heavily timbered area now, even though it was a logging area. When you come out here now, you can barely pick out anything from the 2019 fires; it's completely grown back. We were surrounded by fire; I could sit in my house at night and see an orange glow completely around us.

What I've learned from this experience is that you've got to learn just to be. You learn resilience. At the end of the day, there's the old Paul Keating saying, 'Life's not meant to be easy.'

You can sit down, curl up in a ball, and cry—the flood was very hard on my wife. She's in the fire brigade as well, but she was fine through the fire. As a nurse, she's used to seeing disasters and people in pain.

But the flood hit her fairly hard, so we went away on an extended holiday afterwards. My wife says, 'You're just too laid-back,' but I've never had anyone do anything for me. Ever since I left the army, I've worked for myself, and I wasn't born with a silver spoon in my mouth. I've made my own bed and worked hard my whole life. I've never expected anyone to do anything.

Then, coming to a place like this and seeing people go out of their way to help you in many different ways. People were doing whatever they could. I know I keep harking back to the fires, but the stuff that people were dropping down at the fire shed during those fires, cakes and lasagne, donating chainsaws and the same at the pub. People would say, 'Is there anything we can do? Is there anything I can do?'

You did have some idiots, mainly tourists, who came up, and I think that was what got to my wife more than anything. Some people came up just to have a look, and we were in the middle of trying to clean the place out, and these people pulled up in their little flash Mercedes Benz sports car and wandered across the road. One of them asked a stupid question, I can't even think what it was, but my wife swore at them and told them in no uncertain terms to get out of town.

The people in the area would never do that. The other one was the helping people. People are very quick to bag the council and governments but help and assistance were offered without us asking. Services New South Wales sent people out to check on everyone and that the community hall was above the flood mark. They set up services to go through with people what they're entitled to and what they can do. One was a specialist businessperson. She was very good. We had local members or councillors come out, not too big-note themselves, although I must admit people tend to give them a bit of a hard time. They were generally concerned and wanted to see what they could do to help.

One was our new member in the federal government, a guy named Dan Repacholi. He's big; you can't miss him. He'd only just been voted in, and he's dropped in here a couple of times now. It's a long way out of the way for a busy man, whether he's in Canberra or Cessnock.

I'm not basing it on parties or politics. They're just human beings. It's like any high-profile sportsperson when you get to know some of them. The beauty of living in a community like this is that you already know that about people because you've spoken to them and run into them. We've got one general store in town, two cafes and a pub. That's it. It's pretty hard to avoid people. Even when we go into Cessnock for our shopping, we have to stop about five times to chat with someone from Wollombi.

But I can see Wollombi changing now. Many of the original local people or people have been here a long time. We have quite an aged population, as I mentioned earlier. Now they're just lovely old people. But when you listen to their stories, they were hippies who came up here in the seventies because they could smoke dope and keep out of sight.

Now they're these 70- and 80-year-old people, lovely, sweet old ladies and gentlemen who were once these free-spirited wild people. Unfortunately, what's driving them out of here is health issues. A couple of doctors live around here, but they work elsewhere. To go to the doctor, you have to go to Cessnock at minimum, and to get to a decent hospital, you probably need to go to Sydney or John Hunter.

There's a bit of real estate on the market now, but it's grossly overpriced. But what will drive the next change around here will be a generational change because a relatively high percentage of the population needs access to healthcare.

I hope people move here because they want to live the Wollombi lifestyle, not because they want to change Wollombi. But the cost, I suppose, is stopping that.

It's just a shame. When we first bought here, it was quite achievable to buy around here at a reasonable price. Not necessarily a big house or something; there's a lot for sale at the moment, but not a lot selling. The best example I can give you is the general store, which has been for sale since before COVID.

You're looking for a young family to run a general store that's open seven days a week. But for that general store, they want close to $2 million. You can't buy a house around here for under $1.5 million. What young family trying to get out of Sydney has $3.5-$4 million? That's pretty much a starting point up here.

You'll never hear anyone around here say, 'Oh, the government's got to do something about the flooding.' None of them want to move.

The idea of flood mitigation for a flood like that one in July 2022, even if they built mitigation that would have stopped the flood at the 2007 level, would have gone over it.

You just have to accept that that's what happens here. Many people don't have to live here, but they live here because they love it.

Most houses are built above flood levels. The village is probably the most at risk because it's at the lowest point, but many relatively famous people own property up here, and they've been here for years.

If you believe in the goodness of the human spirit and see it occasionally, it makes these things not so bad in the long term. I'm sure there are plenty of people who are nowhere near as positive as me. There are plenty of people who got quite distraught and possibly permanently damaged by living through the floods.

Everyone has challenges, so it doesn't matter where you go. Living in Sydney, it is challenging to get from one place to another in a reasonable time.

I don't miss that. I love it here; the positives far outweigh the negatives.

MELISSA O'TOOLE

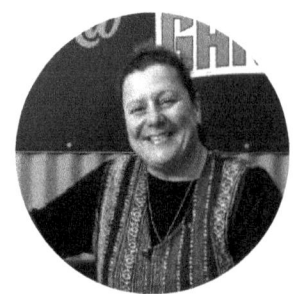

Melissa O'Toole, a well-respected Broke Village local, gives us her perspective on the floods both from her personal experience and from what is now a hub of the village, Magoony's Coffee House, which plays an important part in village life.

Melissa and her husband Paul moved to Broke nearly 30 years ago with their family and ran a couple of businesses. Her husband is a teacher at St Catherine's School in Singleton.

She worked for 18 years in local businesses in the area, including Margan Wines. On their two-acre property on the outskirts of the village, they have a catering business, Motty's Farm Cuisine, and a guest house called Red Tractor Retreat.

They had an antique shop many years ago and took on the old garage where they had planned to open another antique shop but have since turned into a cellar door. Their son Ryan runs the now iconic Magoony's Coffee House in the same location.

Melissa highlights the challenges of rebuilding and finding strength in the face of the devastation caused by the floods and provides outstanding examples of neighbours and volunteers offering assistance and support.

She describes how the community bonded and thrived amidst the challenging circumstances of a natural disaster and how places like the

Broke Village Hall and Magoony's Coffee House enable people to gather and share their experiences and to continue to support those who are still dealing with the aftermath of the floods.

Melissa has a positive but realistic outlook about the future of Broke, where floods are part of the history of their environment.

'I think most likely there will be another flood... a lot of people have got their own views, but I don't have a concern for my future of living here. If it's going to happen, it's going to happen. It was one in a hundred-year flood. Maybe it's another hundred years.'

We had 28 years of all four of our children all attending the little Broke school. They've all ventured out. We told them all to get the hell out of Broke and experience the world; they haven't entirely experienced the world, but they've got out of Broke, and one's come home to run the coffee shop.

The best thing about living in Broke was bringing our children up here and creating lifelong friends. When your children go to school, that's where you meet your long-term friends, which we still have in the area. It's been lovely bringing them up in the country on some land. Growing our own veggies, having a few animals, and just having that country village spirit, which for us took over after the floods.

Because we lived out of town, there were many people we didn't know. Then, with our children going into St. Catherine's College, we lost some more contact, and people came and went. But once the floods hit, we met some very special people and became good friends with them.

Our family home is just on the outskirts of the village. It's on a couple of acres on the Wollombi Brook, so, over the years, we've been used to having the water level come up. The old Broke bridge, across to Milbrodale Road, was a low, rickety bridge, so we'd be cut off, and everyone had to go round the long way to town.

When our four children left home, we turned our family home, which is now called Red Tractor Retreat, into a homestay. We live in a little humpty down in the bush near Wollombi, which we love. The first part of the road that usually goes under flood is the road that heads down to Winmark Wines and Krinklewood towards Wollombi.

On the day of the flood, we had a specialist appointment for Paul in Newcastle that we couldn't cancel. The rain had been coming down heavily for 24 hours, and we wondered if it would go over. We got to Newy, and I remember ringing Kenny in the fire brigade and saying, 'Do you think we'll get back home?'

He said, 'You're gone, you're under. You won't be going back home.'

We thought that was pretty quick. We had some guests checking into the guest house, and we weren't worried about that too much; it's not going to come up. We had the appointment and quickly got back on the phone with Kenny. He said, 'You've definitely gone under; it's coming up quick, Mel.'

We went home to talk to the guests. As we were coming into Broke, there was a floodplain and a lot of flats. We said, 'Oh, my God, look at the water over the road; this is going to go under soon. We've never seen this under water.'

By then, the adrenaline starts settling in a bit, and we wonder how much it's going to come up. It'll still be another 24 hours or two days. We got on Facebook and spoke to people at Wollombi, asking how far it was coming up. Then we went to the guest house, and a van pulled up with two big dogs, four kids, and two ladies. We told them we've got a fair bit of water coming up, but it never floods in Broke. You'll be right.

They got their red wine and were excited, saying, 'We're not going anywhere. We've just come out of COVID. We've been hanging out for this trip.'

We were just going to get settled when Benny, our neighbour, who has a guest house next door, said, 'There's no one in this weekend. You and Paul are cut off, so stay here and just pretend you're having a night away.' We went into town, got some cheese, wine, and goodies, and wondered what was going to happen, how far it was going to come up, and how long it would take.

Then, the SES pulled up. 'You've got to evacuate.'

'No, the water hasn't come up yet.' We walk down the back. On the property, there's a 14-metre drop to the brook. It has only ever lapped the top of the property on the weekend of the Pasha Bulker grounding.

Our guests said, 'She'll be right.' We told them we were in the house next door; we'll keep them posted.

When 3 pm came, the SES said, 'You've got to go.'

We said, 'What are you talking about? Come on, girls. We'll go and walk down the back.'

It was knee-deep, heading towards us. That sent us all into a whirlwind. We've got a granny flat down the back on the brook, and Hugh, who was renting there, had just pulled up saying, 'I've got to start throwing stuff in. I just got to get what I can. It's coming in a bit more.'

We started panicking and said to the guests, 'We've never seen it sort of up like this. Maybe you should get on your merry way.'

They said, 'We've had a couple of bottles of wine; we've just unpacked everything.'

We said, 'Well, put it this way: It's either you pack up now, or we could all be spending the night together in the guest house.'

They all packed up, and believe it or not, we only found out a few hours later that they had headed out on the only road open to Singleton. Within a few minutes of them getting up the road, the road washed away, and the power lines went down.

Then we went down to the new back shed. My dad and Paul's mum had passed away the previous year, and we had a lot of furniture and their belongings down there.

We started lifting everything on top as high as we could, not thinking how fast it would go up or that it would go as far as it did.

Then it started to get dark, and the water was still rising. We were wading through it, still moving. We'd parked the cars down the front of the driveway, which was one of the highest points, and it was just starting to lap on the step to get into my Pajero.

We were edging the car along. We didn't think about an old collector's car that Paul had down the back shed, but it's gone. Then we got into a bit of a kerfuffle and thought, oh my God, this pod down the back hasn't been tied down; it's on piers.

I raced up the fire shed, saying, 'Has anyone got torches? The power has gone out. What are we going to do? We think we're going to lose this pod.' No one knew what was going on and how far the water would go.

We said, 'We don't have torches or anything.' They said, 'Go back home. A lot of the people have already been evacuated on buses. We'll keep going past, up and down, and you'll see the fire truck, and the lights… to reassure you.'

We had a plan next door with Benny. We're pretty close to our neighbours. Benny and Paul said, 'Righto, what's the plan?' Suddenly, I saw ladders going up on one level of the veranda onto the roof.

I said, 'What are you doing?'

Paul said, 'This is the escape plan. You're going to spend the night on the roof if you have to.'

We had to because the water was coming across the paddock and our pool, and we saw we were an island. We decided to wait and see. By this time, it was probably only up half a metre, about five, six o'clock at night. We just put the fire on and settled in. I was in the lounge. Paul was constantly doing the rounds of the veranda. He had a stick and was measuring where the level was going.

I remember by 2 am, it had stopped and lapped the veranda of our main family home.

We have a kids' retreat out the back. It went under a metre. We didn't expect that. Beds, carpet. It went through our pod, a metre, and all our sheds and mowers.

Some of the furniture was saveable, but over the next couple of days, when the water went down, slippers, CDs, shoes, and all sorts of items were caught in the fence between Benny's place and us. But nothing too sentimental was gone.

We managed to save some of Paul's mother's nice furniture. It was up high on some of the tables. But we lost a lot of camping gear and mowers, and God knows what, there were piles and piles of stuff out in front.

We're set back a fair bit from the road, so we only saw what was going on in our front yard. When the water was high, it would have been over my knees, and I'm quite tall. I would walk down the front stairs and hang onto the stair rail, then walk about three metres to grab onto the pool fence because the water was moving so fast towards the road.

Then, to get to the car, we would just hang on to trees. You couldn't walk from the car back to the house without hanging on to things, or you would be knocked over.

It was unbelievable and something I'd never seen before. It was scary. But it was two years ago. I probably don't look scared or upset now, but I remember going down to the fire shed. The adrenaline was pumping the whole way through. I'm a bit like that now, thinking about it. There were many tears.

I remember when the water was coming up in the afternoon after the guests had left. I was on the veranda, just thinking, what am I going to do? What are we going to move? How far is this going to come up? I was not expecting what it did at all. Then I heard this almighty noise from my husband.

His dad died of a heart attack; I've always got that on my mind. It was just in between the shed. Honestly, it was a noise, as if he was having a heart attack. I looked down the back of the trees, and he's got this massive, big going away suitcase made of timber and leather like people used to have on the train trips out west. You packed all your stuff in it.

He's got it almost on his shoulders, nearly killing him, and he's just about crying, going, 'I've got to get this. You've got to help me.' It's got everything from our four children's time at school: all the paintings, report cards, little things they've made, and photos.

I don't know what he was going to do, but no matter what, it got back into the house, on a table, in pride of place. It was not going to get wet.

You wish you could go back and think, could I have done more? We were only discussing that in the car today. He said, 'Why didn't we think about the cars in the shed?' I had an old collector's BMW that wasn't insured, and he's got an old VW Karmann Ghia. There were too many other things to think about, like the cars that we drive every day. I don't know how they didn't get flooded.

At this stage, we had no power, so we had no lights, no mobile phone reception, and no water. We'd managed to have dinner and lit the fire, and that was pretty much us for the night. Knowing that everyone else was in that situation, you were doing what you had to do there and then.

Probably one of the most memorable stories I have is that once the road was opened a week or two down the track, we drove to Wollombi one day and looked up. There's a fridge up in the trees, way above our heads.

There's a bra, there's someone's sheet. Around the village, it was mainly just the grass line and all the paddock stuff. The fence between us and Benny and Jase next door was completely flattened. That's where many of Dad's and Paul's mum's bits and pieces were. We didn't tackle that for a long time. I remember there was so much stuff.

My husband builds tables in his spare time, and we had two big packs of timber, probably 25 -30 metres long, like floorboard timber, and a metre wide, probably a couple of tons. The force of the water moved both of those timber packs a good 50 metres until they just hit a tree. They are still there.

The force was unbelievable. When we went down the back and opened the pod granny flat, it was like it had been tipped upside down. The fridge was upside down. There was a wine fridge, lounge chairs, and beds. I've never seen anything like it in my life. The door was closed, and the water just got in those cracks, and God knows what it did when it was swirling around the force of it.

Many days later, like I said, so much stuff was built up in the fences. But that was something you didn't want to tackle at the time. One day the army people just turned up and said, 'Come on, we're here to help.'

I said to my husband, 'We can't do all this ourselves.' The family had come up and helped us clear out the sheds and put everything out the front like the NRMA had asked us to and rip up the carpet and take the beds out of the retreat, but we couldn't think about the stuff in the paddocks and up against the fences.

But these 20 men were here, and they went in and cleared out the fences and all the debris and tried to help us, which was great.

We were still in the guest house and couldn't return to the property for seven to ten days. We live on the side of a mountain, so it doesn't flood, but the driveway got very wet.

I have a funny story. When we did go down there, I remember driving up the driveway. Quite a few weeks beforehand, we'd had a lot of rain as well. We had a pile of blue metal delivered. I decided to drive around the blue metal like I had done before this amount of rain, thinking this would be all right.

I tried my hardest to drive it backward and forward, put some rocks under it, and tried to reverse out, but I was dead stuck. I thought, oh geez, I'm in trouble, so I raced up to the house and got a bottle of wine. I'll have a couple of glasses because I'm in big trouble.

My husband comes home in his old Land Rover, and I'm sitting on the deck looking down at him on the driveway coming up, and he does exactly what I did. He drives up to the metal, goes back, and thinks, I'll go around. He went around, and he sank right next to me. We had both cars sunk in the mud, and we had to get Adrian, a mate in town who has an excavating business. 'Mate, can you come and help us? Can you come and pull us both out? We're both bogged.'

Unfortunately, we lost all our food in the fridge. But nothing down there; it was mainly the family home and guest house.

It was very sad driving around, seeing good friends, a couple of families in particular, with a house full of kids and all of their belongings on the side of the road. That was the hard thing in the village. We're a tourist town, and we didn't have accommodation bookings for quite a few months while we were trying to clean up. But that was the least of our worries.

We didn't want anyone in the town coming in, looking at everything, and being in the way. We wanted to cocoon where the main hub was. The best thing out of it, for me, was how this hub became the local meeting point at the hall where Monkey Place Catering was set up, and we all went down there and we'd do rosters. I'd go next door and help Jase. She had a little boy, and she was pregnant. 'What do you need, Jase? Let's get in and do some prep and help out.'

We'd take turns and had a roster serving the food. Everyone went there. You went down there, and you'd just sit there, and there'd be a young woman on a chair with the kids, just thinking. Someone would be talking to someone else they haven't talked to for a while. 'Wow, are you going? What do you need?'

There was a man who lived in a caravan park down the road near where I live now. I've never met him before but still see him in our coffee shop. He'd just sit there; he wanted to be a part of things. It was so nice. Every day, he was there waiting to light up the barbecue or serve the sausages. I got to know people I've never known in 20 years in the village. Although many people stuck to themselves and some older people had their own set of friends, there was camaraderie and pulling together of all the different people who lived in Broke and their stories.

We were supposed to open the coffee shop around the time the floods hit. We didn't get much damage here. The house next door was flooded, so we got a lot of runoff. We mainly had mud to clean up. But we thought this was not the time to open, and we were all struggling. Many people were struggling much more than we were and didn't have houses to live in, so we put the opening on the back burner for September.

The meeting place was in the hall for about a month. You'd get up and say, 'Come on, let's go down.' I'd go down at least every day to have a chat, have a coffee, and help with the catering; it was almost like medicine.

You'd go inside the hall if you needed clothes or food. There was a board with a list of which houses were going to have the pump-out system done, who had a sinkhole, and who needed this. It just shows you what a village is all about. That's what got a lot of people through.

Of course, that couldn't go on forever. We'd never intended for this coffee shop to be such a social hub for locals, but people were like, 'Oh, how are you going, Johnny? Hey, Betty, how are you?' And it's still like that nearly two years down the track. Bob will come out of the bush that lives on his own and does his own thing, and he'll sit on the end of the table in his seat for two hours. It's just so lovely to be a part of, to continue that because in Broke, there are cellar doors and a couple of restaurants, there's the Broke village store, but there was nowhere like a coffee shop where people can just come and sit and watch people come and go and chat to them if they want or leave when they want.

The timing was unbelievable. I think it's helped some people through it. A couple of families still aren't in their house, and back then, when the coffee shop opened, they spent a lot of time here. They can come and go when they want, but it was still somewhere for a bit of network and support, 'Are you all right today, mate? Do you need a hand or some food, or do you need a hand with that? How's it all going?' We've been very fortunate.

I think many people are still suffering. You don't know because we still don't see much of the community in the coffee shop. Not everyone is a coffee drinker or wants to come and talk to people, and everyone's got their own life and is busy, so I don't know how everyone's getting on. But about a month ago, we had the first big rain since the floods, and it brought a lot of raw feelings back.

The other day, I was talking to Robbie, Mike, and a couple of others and asked, 'How'd you go the last couple of weeks?' We all said it brought everything back.

Recently, I was talking to Kathleen, who ran the fire shed and helped me with the guest house, and she said, 'What do you reckon about this rain, Mel?'

I said, 'I don't know. I reckon the brook's coming up again. It could get us down at the bottom.' You're not thinking that this will ever happen again. We hope not in our lifetime.

Kathleen said, 'I've got a meeting with the SES.' We both stood there and teared up, hanging on for a minute. Is this going to happen again? No, not yet. It's not even two years.

Some people aren't yet in their houses, and others have just gotten by. I don't know if people could get through if it happened again so quickly.

We've got the warning system in place now, and its Mother Nature. We had the fires, and that wasn't as bad because it was a slow burn, and you could see it. We live on the mountain, and we had our mountain burn behind us within a couple of metres of our house, but you could monitor it.

Whereas I remember asking Kathleen what about this? She said, 'I'd rather fight a fire than a flood because it's all the cleaning up afterward.'

As I said, our fences are still down between Benny and us after nearly two years, although we're getting them done now. But the piles of timber are still there, and there's stuff that I don't know if we'll ever fix up. Probably the worst thing was our pool, which was half full of sand from the brook. It was unbelievable. I'd never seen anything like it in my life—the amount of sand that came out of that brook, the destruction.

We have our pool back, but it took a long time. I've got a brother-in-law who's a pool man, and he fixed it. The water wasn't drained out of it; they put stuff in and vacuumed it, and we got new pumps. Everything had to be replaced.

If I think about what I learned from the flood, it was that if something bad happens and you need to pull together, there are people here. We've got a Broke notice board online, and I've noticed it more so since the floods. If someone needs something or wants something on there, bang. What do you need? Where do you need it? We'll be there. I can remember someone saying, 'We need a hand with pulling someone's spa out,' and bang, there will be five blokes there. Living here for so long, we've never really needed that community support.

I have to say, living in Broke, I want to live near the beach in the summer. But now autumn's hit, and I'm not going anywhere. We live in a special part of the world. There are a lot of special people here in Broke.

You go back to sticking to yourself and doing your own thing, and you're busy; if I needed someone or anyone out there needed a hand, there will be people knocking on the door or knocking the door down to help you. That's the biggest thing.

We see that a lot here in the coffee shop. People come here to talk. I'm Ryan's mum, and it's his business, but Paul and I are often here having a chat and seeing how people are. People tell you all their stuff because you're here, and you're the front of the face of the place. Sometimes, you just don't know what people are going through.

I never thought I would be a part of living here, but from being part of it, I realised good things came out of it—being part of the community that we are, with everyone pulling together. The services that we were offered were the biggest piece of support that we had. We got so much help here from so many different people and services. We were so fortunate, but I wouldn't want it to happen again to anyone.

What impressed me was people helping others rather than putting themselves first. Like the people in the fire brigade, their houses were going under. They had families at home but were doing their jobs and volunteering. A handful of people were there day by day, just getting out of bed, helping everyone try to get by and sort out their houses and what was going on, not worrying about what was going on at home. That blew a lot of people away; just selfless.

You've got the voluntary services; that's what they have to do. But so many other people stepped up. We were all in it together. What do you need doing? We can organise this or that to be done.

As time goes by—it's been nearly two years—it's a shame that something like that has to happen to show people what we're like. But as I said, if tomorrow something bad happens again, bang, those same people will be there.

I like giving and helping. I'm a giver, not a taker. I enjoy nurturing and fussing over people. The floods also broadened my eyes to what a great little community we have. I'm proud to say Broke's where I live. But I wouldn't like to go through it again.

We're a tight little community. We are bringing more activities to the hall. There's a small group doing that. It will be nice to see more things. Not everyone can get to them during the week, but I'd love to see a bush dance on a Friday night or use the hall more, which Evelyn's trying to do. But more community things are happening, which is great.

We've got the Bicentennial coming up soon, which we'll all be a part of, and things like the Broke Village fair. Broke is also a tourist destination. There are always things happening.

A couple of different things will always remind us of the floods. Because of where we live, we're always down the back checking the creek's level. Has it come up? There are even things still stuck in the fence.

I don't think about it much, but I went down the back to see Ryan's pod to get his dog and saw someone digging a hole. It's getting fixed. Then I walked past the bits of timber and thought they might get moved back to where they belonged one day.

But they'll always be memories. The back toilet out the back is always blocked, probably full of mud, and we have never got it to work since the floods. There are a few things that'll never be the same.

There was a smell that had been around for a long time, but what was heartbreaking was seeing everyone's belongings on the side of the road after people had cleared out their houses.

There are a couple of empty houses on Wollombi Street, which you see every day. There's one house down near me that's still got the fencing around it. I heard the other day that it's about insurance problems or something. Recently, one house I know of in the village was bulldozed and is now a vacant block of land. There are still memories around that are there in front of you.

I don't think about the future of Broke too much. I believe tourism will continue; people will move into the area. Some of us thought people would stay away and not buy here after hearing about the floods. We'll keep moving along; you can't control Mother Nature. I don't even know exactly how the warning systems work.

We've had a fair few floods where the roads have been shut in my time. But with these floods, the water came from every direction. I have my theory, thinking maybe bushfires cleared away everything, and we had so much downpour that it just came out of the mountains.

But when you go to people's houses over the years, we've all got different views. It's such a pretty place. Mike, who lives on the flats, said, 'I've never seen water come from behind me. Like it just came from all directions.' I'm not worried about living in Broke and Wollombi for the future.

I think, most likely, there will be another flood. There are a lot of trees in the brook that we say shouldn't be there and haven't been there for the whole of the hundred years. People have their own views, but I am not concerned about living here for my future. If it's going to happen, it's going to happen. It was one in a hundred-year flood. Maybe it's another hundred years. Let's hope it's not like Lismore, with quite a few in a short period, but who knows?

I hope we move on and the people still not in their homes get into them soon. I hope we don't have too many more raw memories when we have a downpour and that we continue going the way we are. We don't need too many more changes here. Hopefully, we continue as a community and come together in other ways than when we're dealing with a flood or a fire.

It was just normal people doing their everyday things, and then bang! But it's getting back to normal now.

I'm fortunate that I get to see that here in the coffee shop. You get to keep in touch with the regulars, and it's good.

KIRSTY & QUINTON MCCLEOD

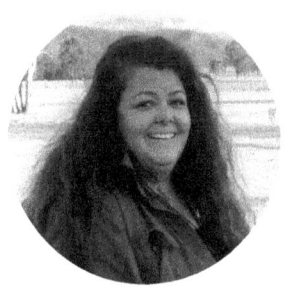 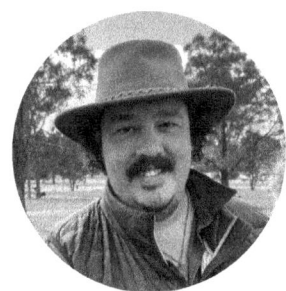

Kirsty and Quinton McCleod are the couple who manage Starline Alpacas Farm stay in Broke.

They have a shared passion for farming, agritourism, and the growth and development of the region.

Quinton came to the region with an interest in viticulture, but his farming background saw him return to his first love, and alpacas took the limelight.

Kirsty, who has a criminology background, saw her work pivot in a rural setting, where she fell in love with the idea of making the farming experience and tourism accessible to everyone.

During the devastating floods on the 6th of July 2022, they used their resources to shelter as many families as possible. Having kids of their own, they recognised the importance of having a space for kids to feel moments of normality and safety away from flood waters while their parents navigated rebuilding their lives. Along with some incredible local educators, they were able to provide a space for a play group.

Kirsty and Quinton share their insights and observations of the devastating flood's impact on Broke and the residents following some rough years of drought, fire, and the pandemic.

Their love for their community shines through their words, and so does their strong belief in the future of this unique town in the Hunter region.

Kirsty: How we came to live in Broke is an interesting story. With a criminology and social science background, I have spent a lifetime trying to be a helping person. I helped a young person who said to me, 'I want to give something back to you. I want to gift you a holiday as a thank you for my life.'

Quinton: We had met and married in the region, and when we came up for the holiday; it was our first chance to get away since our son was born. At the time, I was working as a chemical formulator for a company on the Central Coast. It was quite dangerous and wasn't great for my health. I'd had enough.

Previously, I had worked on farms, but while visiting wineries in the area, I decided to ask people if they had work. Two weeks later, I had a job in a winery. I was doing all their tractor and vineyard work, and that's how we got into the valley.

After doing that for four years, I was offered the farming position here at Starline and never looked back.

Kirsty: We've become very passionate about this life and have combined some of our skills and knowledge into a weird concoction of agritourism management with alpacas.

Quinton: It was also the fact that we both grew up in cities and didn't want that for our kids. I wanted them to be more countryfied and learn hands-on things rather than being in the city, and this ticked all the boxes for us.

Once we looked into agritourism and how it worked, we realised we could give that country experience to the city folk and let them know what it is like out here.

Kirsty: An interesting fact about our moving here is that I'd got dressed for our wedding here in Broke. Later, I found out that some of my relatives were among the first settlers of Broke, so I've come home after a long and convoluted life.

Back to place, back to land—that is our goal in our vision for Starline. We've chosen to make it about the morals we have for country hospitality, inclusivity, and passion. We love the old way of doing things, so we have spinning and fibre. We've got mindfulness and healing workshops and community programs.

We also had outdoor day care, like a rewilding program, for a time because it's something a little lost.

Quinton: Getting people away from technology and back into hands-on and feeling things and looking at things from a different perspective.

Kirsty: Many people go to the supermarkets for their groceries but have no idea where things come from.

Now, we're not technically in the market for producing food or vegetables yet, but we've produced a fibre that is quite good for things like jumpers. People buy woollen jumpers from a store, and they're expensive because it's a good product, but they don't understand where it comes from.

They don't understand what it means to raise an animal and make sure that everything is nice and healthy to give us the products we use daily. It's a great passion for us to give other people coming to the farm the opportunity to see that.

Quinton: On July 6th, the day of the flood, eight families were on the site, including our family.

Kirsty: In the days before the flood, I had been preparing. I've always had what I call a country woman's knowingness. I had been preparing for something, and preparedness is very much in my nature.

Maybe a week before, I was even saying to Quinton, 'I think you need to go get petrol.'

He said, 'Why would I need to do that?'

I replied, 'Because I'm telling you.'

Which is such a blessing because we had some. I'm very much into the homesteading culture, so we were already at a level of preparedness, which was of benefit in the immediate situation.

Quinton: We had cupboards full of food and were prepared for what would happen. We're situated up high, but the flooding came in very quickly, it came much faster than most people thought it would.

Kirsty: In the lead-up, we were listening to things including some of the old knowledge. Some people were saying, 'Nah, it's not going through.' But some of our older generation remembered the stories from a little while ago and said, 'Look, it is a possibility.' I took that to be that I'm going to trust the old knowledge. We were moving the alpacas to the highest ground.

Quinton: We're quite lucky, given the fact that we are up on a hill. Although it's not a very big hill, we ended up being an island on the street.

We're fortunate that we had a large backup solar system. Our function centre and four cottages are all off-grid. We were able to put the families into the off-grid cottages. They were from Sydney and other cities, so they weren't used to having no power or running water; out here, it's all tank water.

Kirsty: Our concern was knowing the resources and preparedness, and our level of knowledge was good; how could we get our community to our place? This is in our skill set; all the off-grid stuff, different modes of cooking, and generators. Preparedness is a passion for us.

Quinton: Since the flood, we've also informed the town's local services that we have the resources. They were all down at Broke Hall during the flood with no power. They had whiteboards up, saying where everybody was going.

We've also said we're quite happy to house the emergency services because we have an amazing space, solar panels, and power backup to host these people who go out and look after the everyday people.

Kirsty: My background is in high trauma, so I have a skill set that I have to offer: helping identify trauma and helping identify people who are not seeing it. People tend to come to me because they know my history and what I've dealt with. I'm that person, 'the eternal mother', Quinn often calls me. I was preparing to use my grit and deep emotional understanding.

What I didn't prepare for was the gravity of that for me. I don't think either of us ever thought about ourselves until far after the fact. We were like, 'Okay, this is what we can do. This is what we have. These are our strengths. How can we apply that to our community?'

Quinton: We were also prepared for the worst for our animals and other animals, but we didn't expect it to be as bad as it was.

We took it day by day. If you get caught up in the weeds, it won't help you or others. I was lucky enough to get two families from Broke up before the floods, and they stayed on the farm with us. One of them is a good friend, and he helped me carry hay bales across the floodwaters to people's horses stuck out in Broke.

Getting out once the flood had receded enough for us to cross was almost like a mini-war zone. It was quite surreal to walk around and see how bad it was and how badly the damaged places were.

Kirsty: I think the harder part for us was that when you're talking about emotional preparedness, when you are directly affected but indirectly as well, you don't have the same level of adrenaline going as other people do. It becomes like compassion fatigue.

When you're going through something, when you're in it, it's practical. But looking at it from the outside, it's quite shocking to observe many people's experiences. I felt an overwhelming empathy for them.

Quinton: When I managed to get into town to try and help people out, Kirsty had messaged me that quite a few people were evacuated. Suddenly, my phone went off, saying, 'Can you go to my house? I didn't get a chance to lock it up. There's looting going on. Can you please go look up this?

Check out the house. Let me know if there's any damage.'

Things like that happened. Although, at the time, I didn't think much of it. I went in and locked people's houses up for them. When you sat back and thought about it, who would loot an area that's been destroyed?

Kirsty: To be honest, I was hoping you didn't meet any of them face-to-face because I don't know how that would go.

Quinton: I was there during daylight hours; plenty of people around us with the SES and others.

It was devastating going onto people's properties and through their houses; walking through some people's flooded houses, then some people's houses weren't even touched.

Kirsty: Nothing can prepare you for that because these are not strangers. They are school mums. They're mates you've had a beer with. They're the people you've been there for with other losses, or their little kids' birthday parties.

These are families where you've supported their business, and they've supported you. In a rural community, our lives are intertwined in a way, and our livelihoods are intertwined in a different way, so the effects are more personal. Whether or not it directly happened to you, as a community, it has a very deep impact.

Quinton: Broke is a community where everyone knows everyone. There are families that have been here for 100 years, and all their kids, grandkids, and great grandkids have gone through public school.

Then there are people like us who come to the community and are welcomed with open arms because we not only care but also help out; it's the, 'You scratch my back; I'll scratch your back' mentality. We've lived on the Central Coast, in Sydney, and in places like that, where you often don't know your neighbours.

Kirsty: But here you do. In a way, what's theirs is yours, so you care about their property, animals, kids, and family. Leading up to the flood, our mindset was, how will we get people out with mobility issues or people who are struggling? We knew one local person who'd recently gone through a separation; did she have the skills? Could she get her animals out and load them? We were thinking of what we could do and how much we could bring in.

Quinton: Our house can get flooded; yes, we're affected, but nothing like how they were affected in the town. Although we didn't have power in our house, we had power on the farm.

We were able to go into town and offer help and accommodation. We tried everything that we could to help others because it wasn't about us at all; it was about what we could do to help people who we've grown to appreciate and respect.

Kirsty: We could offer dry firewood, which we did for anybody who needed that. Those were the things that were appreciated. I have a beautiful local friend, Beth, who struggled to keep her kids warm. She said to me, 'The best thing for me was that firewood so I could keep my children warm.'

The first thing I noticed is people out here are usually self-reliant. I often heard, 'Oh, there's someone worse off than me.' I said, 'I don't want to offend you here, but you are that person who needs help right now.'

Quinton: I think it is an Australian way to do that. I went into a lady's house. I'm six feet two inches, and the water level was up to my shoulders.

Kirsty: I remember she fell into my arms. I told her, 'You're not okay,' so I sent Quinton over. You're so stoic, but…

Quinton: I went there and talked to them, saying, you can come and stay on the farm. We have power. You can be close to your house. You can spend your day there and come back to a warm shower. Many people said, 'I'm not doing that. I'm not leaving the house.'

They are strong people out here—hats off to them—and they push through it.

We could do little things like get a heater out to somebody. Because we run a farm stay, I've got contacts for air conditioning and electricals and stuff like that. We called our contacts to come and check on people's houses to see if they can get things running properly for them.

Little things like that were big for them.

Kirsty: We tried to keep it very quiet. It's the first time I've ever spoken about it. Because for us, it was not about anyone knowing. We wanted to maintain everyone's privacy and help out in the way that we could. We set up food supplies for anyone on-site. I would put food out every day for them.

Quinton: We also turned our function centre into a kindergarten, like a day care for all.

Kirsty: We are a family establishment with a lot of knowledge about kids and floodwaters.

Quinton: The local teachers came out and helped with the day care. While the parents were dealing with the flooding, the kids were at least in a safe environment and able to play and have a little bit of normality before going back to a flood-affected house.

Kirsty: We were a bit worried, knowing what kids are like and that they won't understand the gravity of flood water. Not everyone thinks about it. 'Oh, it's a bit of water.'

Well, it's not a little bit of water in a flood.

Quinton: Most houses in town and out here are on septic tanks. All of that went under, but people don't realise that. It's not something you want to be stuck in.

There was a massive effort from the SES and even the local mines. They sent out people to help. We don't compare to what they did, or the RFS, who went around helping other people before they helped themselves. What we did was small in comparison to all those services and water truck volunteers and all that stuff.

Kirsty: We were one little cog in the big wheel of things. When we think now about how it affected the community and what we learned, I don't think it will ever quite be the same. You've got to see the best. I don't want to say the worst, but the best of the worst of people in stress, in trauma, in the way people respond.

You got to see the people that were wanting to help. Some people would shut down. They all had a different coping strategy.

As we touched on earlier, a tiny few in the community were opportunistic. I got to learn the character of many people. There are some inspiring stories. I learned how important it is to live in a community like this, how that's been a little bit lost in some places, and how fortunate we are to have a community that will band together. Hats off to Mick McCardle! (See Mick's story)

Quinton: His response was incredible, and it was so hard for him, and he is going through his own stuff. He did a good job as the frontman of the recovery and a local community member. What a leader to have in Broke, someone who will pull themselves together and ignite others.

Kirsty: We saw many people going through their own stuff but being generous for the greater good, like Ev (See Evelyn Hardy's story), who did the most amazing job. She's an incredible local. I call her Broke's matriarch. She did a fantastic job pulling together at the Broke Hall.

I also want to touch on what I learned about what's important to people. When anyone is dealing with a rural community, they need to understand that the concept of family is different out here. It's not the person's family unit; it's the neighbours. It's the animals.

Some of these animals and the genetics that farmers have been working on are so old and important. They are livelihoods. That's included in the concept of family out here.

Quinton: You've got to look at the animal side of things. When you're dealing with a flood or a fire, you have to open the gates and say, 'Sorry, guys, but this is the best I can do.'

I hope to God that they get out and can fend for themselves because if we have flooding on this farm, we've got close to 90 alpacas. There's no way I would be able to move all of them. It's the same with a lot of people out here with animals and cattle.

Also, the vineyards. All that water would have destroyed all the grapes. It's been a few tough seasons out here. From drought to fires to flooding, that's three seasons lost.

Kirsty: Broke as a town has been through the drought, then the fire. There's a lot of smoke damage on the grapes. Then, the pandemic, and now we've had a flood. In terms of resilience and gravity, how many hits can a community take when it relies on tourism and farming?

Quinton: The community's resilience is astounding, and we still have people in town who aren't in their houses.

Kirsty: One of my best friends in town, is finally nearly at the stage of having her house rebuilt. And this has now been going on for a long time.

Quinton: Much of it has to do with insurance and things like that.

Kirsty: There is also the legacy that the floods left in rebuilding livelihoods because our livelihoods out here are intertwined with the country, the land, and tourism. The tourism sector has taken a hit, our landscape has taken a hit, and animals and our families have taken a hit.

'Broke broke me.' I kind of get that when some people say it.

Quinton: I think it's grit and determination. You have to stop and walk outside with your cup of coffee in the morning, and look at your backyard and say, 'That's why we're here.' You see the mountain range. You don't hear the cars. This is why we're here.

Kirsty: We do it for our neighbours, too. If you give up, there is a flow-on effect. If we gave up, the weddings would get lost. We are the largest accommodation venue in the region. That would go away. The tourist traffic goes away if you give up. That's why I mentioned the importance of community. It has an effect, and you don't want to be the weak one amongst all these strong people.

Quinton: The businesses in Broke are all part of an ecosphere. We all contribute to tourism. People come and look at the alpacas, or they go to the different vineyards or the local shop. If one of us falls down, then tourism and the economy of the area will suffer.

Kirsty: I can't imagine many Broke people giving up. If you've got that attitude, you'll fit in here great.

Out here, there, and in most rural communities, you'll know that there are extra support services for mental health. We have lost members, which is very sad.

Quinton: We've also got to stop being hardarses.

Kirsty: We do.

Quinton: I know down at the Broke Hall, and I haven't gone yet, but they do a cup of tea and a chat once a month. Having that open discourse, being able to say, 'Look, I'm struggling. I need help,' and being willing to accept that help. Whether it is for mental health or someone coming to fix the fence for you.

Kirsty: People are more likely to accept help from a neighbour; the response on the ground after the flood was good. I remember talking to a lady called Tabitha, and she said, 'I'm telling you that you're going to crash. I can see it in you because you keep going.'

The support services were good, and they need to be continued. I know Mick was very good about putting those support services out there. We facilitated, with some fantastic local ladies, to get some grants happening, and we provided the venue for the BRCA and some yoga teachers to get together and create a wellness group.

Quinton: We host a weekly yoga class, and they also do kids' yoga.

Kirsty: Some other healing things were put into place to rebuild wellness. We've tried to offer a place for locals to come and practice mindfulness. We have sound healing and ice baths also happening in the space.

I think any investment in a community's wellness and recovery is worth it, especially in a community like this one that's had several big hits. I don't know if you look at statistics, but in rural communities, the men don't have enough places to go. Men out here are even more stoic than most.

Quinton: I'm guilty; I think most blokes are. We're not a talkative bunch and we don't wear our feelings on our sleeves. The guys out here are all hardworking miners and farmers.

I think we're trying to figure out a way for guys to get together and sometimes not even talk about their feelings, but have another bloke to talk to, like the Men's Shed.

Kirsty: The beautiful Bianca has an idea about having a Men's Shed, working with Soldier On, and providing a space for some of that healing work to happen.

Quinton: From my point of view, when I'm having a bad day or down on myself, I do something physical, whether it is fencing, building a table, or dealing with the animals, and it all goes away. It's our natural way of coping, giving you that break to think about things.

It was hard to watch the effect of the flood on people's lives.

When you were walking or driving the streets, it took a while before we could get a vehicle in there.

A friend of mine crossed the flood water with a long stick, and he told me where there were holes while I was carrying a bale of hay to feed some horses. A young lady was in tears because her horse wouldn't load. She had recently separated and didn't have anyone there to help her.

Quinton: After the floodwaters receded and we managed to get back out of town, the whole interior of every house was out in front.

Kirsty: Some even had signs on them, which was the hardest part, saying, 'Please don't take these,' so at least the assessors can look at it.

It was like a council clean-up, where people go and pick through your rubbish. Many people, especially at night, would drive around and pick through people's trash. They call it disaster tourism.

Quinton: Then, all the businesses got together and said, 'To keep the economy going, we're going to stay closed for this period, then we're going to start opening back up.' That was because we didn't want to bring the tourists into the area and for people to have that privacy to grieve.

Kirsty: People lost their photos of loved ones; even people who'd lost a child lost every photo record.

We went to one of the meetings in the church, and a lady stood up in the middle of the meeting and said, 'I found someone's ashes.' Ashes were floating around, and we did not know who they belonged to.

All the people's lives and all the kids' toys were contaminated. People must have felt so invaded and vulnerable that they lost everything.

Quinton: Some of the stories that came out were devastating. Not being able to find your pets, your animals. You're losing everything. You can't truly comprehend the gravity of the loss. It's not the immediate loss. It's the loss of everything you've treasured and then rebuilding. But it's not the same. Then it's the loss of your future such as a crop or livestock. It's so big. Driving through, it was very much like a war zone.

Kirsty: Some of the people were kind of shell shocked.

Quinton: Some of the houses had their footings wiped away. There was a caravan in a hole that was as deep as the caravan.

Kirsty: Unfortunately, there was no warning to move into a safe place. Trying to convince some people, especially in a 'She'll be right,' community, was quite a task.

Quinton: On the night of the flood, I was watching the water rise and rise. Then the SES came and said that if you're not out within, I think it was, like, 10 or 15 minutes, you're not leaving the town because the way out was going to get flooded in. That's when I pulled the families aside and offered a place up in the farm. Get your stuff together. Pack your cars. Let's go.

Quinton: When I first went into town before the flood happened, there was no water over the bridge. As I came back out to come back to the farm, it was lapping the bottom of my 4WD ute.

Kirsty: You were probably one of the last out.

Quinton: I managed to get a couple of families across. A lot of the other people had already evacuated with buses.

Kirsty: We have been asked if any good came out of this experience? One good thing that came out of this was you got to know people in the community at a level that you didn't previously.

Quinton: It definitely brought community together. It also showed who is a good leader within the community. Who is willing to highlight everyone's skill, put their own stuff aside and then go, okay, I'm willing to help you.

It may be a cliché, but you got to see the good, the bad, and the ugly of the community.

Kirsty: There were some very inspiring and moving stories. You got to see who was willing to be an amazing human and make a difference.

Quinton: At the end of the day, it wasn't about us one particular person. It was about everybody.

Kirsty: It was a coming together in a collective fire. It was a collective rebuild. The Broke Hall became such a hub. You walked in there and you'd see these steel magnolias, ladies who were like, 'Right, I can do food,' so they were doing food. Other people said, 'Okay, I can't do food, but I can do time,' and they were packing grocery things. Local olive producers, Ben and Jace from Monkey Place, offered oil.

Ben was incredible with the catering. He didn't stop for days. He was there at breakfast, like such a shining light in what he did. We provided accommodation if you needed somewhere to stay. We were washing… I can't tell you how many loads of washing. It's what we could do at that moment.

You got to see some of the greatest side of humanity, and that was beautiful.

Another thing we learned was identifying resources for community. We put our hands up and said, 'If anything like this happens again, we have solar, we have paddocks. We could run a hub here. You could have a working commercial kitchen on-site to provide for emergency services.'

Broke has now developed resilience teams for emergencies. There are six of us who are team leaders. We're one of them here, and they're spread out through Broke.

What they found was that everybody in the area was trying to contact the Hall to get information, and they couldn't access it because of all of congestion. Now we've got our resilience team leaders within community so, if something like this happens again, we will have all the information so people can contact us or ask us questions.

The need for advanced warning systems was also recognised. It needs to be advanced because a lot of farmers won't leave their animals. We won't leave our neighbours. You don't leave someone behind, so we need more time to get out because of those factors. It's your livelihood, your family security, your life's work.

Quinton: When it comes to the animals, the farmers are responsible with their animals, so all have to be tagged, for biosecurity reasons as well. If you're going through a disaster where you've had to open your gates up to let them free, you need to locate them again. They need to be correctly tagged so the local land council can pick up the animal and bring it back to them.

Quinton: Then there's the wisdom of the traditional owners of the land who know these areas more than us. There's also the wisdom of the bushcraft people, who know how to use knives and flip flops and all those things to create a fire.

The farmers have their knowledge. There's a collective knowledge there and old wisdom from every corner that you look at when there's no power or no technology. If you're stuck somewhere and you've got no gas, how are you going to start a fire?

Kirsty: I would love to see every family have the capacity to go off grid if the occasion calls for it. We have three months of food ready, so I guess we've learned the importance of being prepared, early intervention, procedures, and now our advanced warning systems coming along in Broke.

Quinton: It all needs to be brought into a collective knowledge base and getting people together to learn that knowledge. I feel that we've lost our way of teaching, it's all done online, and computer-based. There's no hands-on teaching. We've got great people in the area and throughout Australia to hold seminars to teach people the hands-on things they need to know to get through a situation like this.

Kirsty: I love this place. It's quirky, a little bit left of centre, it's got its own vibe. In a way, we're living the dream.

Quinton: I think Broke has got a great future once you get through all that stuff. It's an upcoming region and I see Broke going from strength to strength. As Kirsty was saying, we've gone through a lot from 2019 through to today, with drought, bushfires, COVID, flooding.

Kirsty: I think it's made us stronger as a as a community and as a collective.

Quinton: It's also made us look at what's important and that we need to grow not only as individuals, but as a region and as businesses as well.

Kirsty: We're quite formidable now as a region. What we do need is people to come and visit a wounded community. Please come and support these businesses to get back on their feet. I know you could go to some of our neighbouring regions, but it's important to support the people who've endured. You will be blessing people who need it, and it will be good for your soul to do something like that. I believe if there was ever a town that needed that, it's this one! It makes a difference.

Quinton: Look at the small businesses that are in the area. We've got the soap maker. It's like a little apothecary shop. Now we've got a guy that makes honey mead.

Kirsty: We've got new boutique cellar doors like Cael's Gate coming up, and Hunter Lavender Farm, Magoony's Coffee House, and all the other businesses which have been resilient and need the support to rebuild.

Quinton: If people want to support us and come out to the region, I think they'll realise why we love it. The landscape itself is quite unique, with the mountain range at the back of us.

Kirsty: I know there's some big hotels and fancy overseas things. But, if you could do something in your backyard and support a farmer. I don't think you'd be disappointed with Broke, our quirky little town.

KIRSTY & QUINTON MCCLEOD

TONY HAWKINS

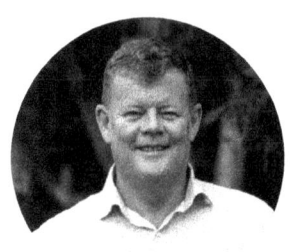

Tony is a long-time resident of the Wollombi area. He moved there with his partner in 1992.

He is a bushfire consultant. If you build in a bushfire-prone area, you'll need a report from somebody like him to assess the risk and determine what you need to do to submit to the council.

For the last few years, he has been involved with training, including in cultural burning practices in the Hunter. Following the fires in 2019, he has been involved in community resilience training.

His story concerns the 2022 Broke and Bulga and Wollombi flood situation. He has a unique perspective and valuable insights because of his long association with the Rural Fire Service (RFS) and community support.

During floods, the community reaches out for help and support from existing community organisations.

I've lived here for over 30 years now. I joined the RFS on the condition that I would not get a position of responsibility, but it wasn't long before they made me a captain. I enjoyed it, and although it was challenging, I later worked for the RFS as a staff member for about eight or nine years.

Wollombi is an interesting place. It's pretty isolated physically, and when events like floods happen, the RFS is the only emergency service in the area, so the RFS is called on to support floods.

I've done a lot of work over the years, and 2007 was also a big flood. But mostly, it's the recovery work. There's not much you can do to hold the water back, is there?

If I had my choice of natural disaster, I would take fire over flood anytime because the cleanup after a flood is heartbreaking and long. The water gets in everywhere, and it's often never the same.

In 2022, the council provided us with many skip bins, which were continually filled with appliances and furnishings. I thought maybe unnecessarily, but most of it you can't recover. It's easier to throw it away.

The 2019 fires were relentless and very different from previous fires. It's the first time I've felt scared because we never seemed to get control of those fires. The chaos or semi-chaos went on day after day. Nothing we did to stop the fires worked.

It took a little while to get over that, and it has certainly affected me since then. After that, we had a bit of relief. A couple of small floods, which were almost welcome after having been dry for so long. Then we got a big one in 2022.

That was very tense. We were all sharing through messages, watching the flood levels, wondering just how high they would go. We were rapidly approaching the record. I only have a little experience with floods in Broke, but I was shocked at what happened there as it was always a place that didn't flood. When it did, it blew my mind.

The area from Wollombi through to Bulga and then down the river was impacted. The famous tavern was underwater.

When I was in the RFS, I felt a responsibility to do what I could, but that was very limited when the flood was coming. I remember, on a few occasions, in floods before 2022, I warned people who were new to the area and living on the flood plain.

During the flood, there's not much you can do. In 2007, we played a minor part in organising people's rescue. But in 2022, it was a matter of waiting until the water level dropped so we could get in and do things. When the water level dropped in the village, particularly at the tavern, it was 'all hands on deck' for whoever could get there.

Only a limited number of people could get there. You do what you can to help people out. In 2022, and this might be controversial, there was a disconnect between the official agencies and the community.

One member of the RFS could access the fire shed and bring a tanker down into the village. He was told he shouldn't be doing that because the SES hadn't tasked him to do that.

Thankfully, he had the courage and strength of character to say no. There was a job to be done, and he did it. It's not a criticism; they're just doing their job. When the SES did turn up after a couple of days, they told us to stop work because they needed to do a risk assessment before we could do any work.

I said, 'Well, hang on. We've been doing this for two or three days. If there's any risk, we've found it and mitigated it.' That sort of thing is frustrating, but it's just the process and can't be helped.

We had people who weren't on the official list for assistance. You ignore the official agencies and go and help them.

Fortunately, a friend had left his bobcat with me for safekeeping. I'd done about three days of work helping people with things like mattresses. The massive skips they sent us had 12-foot sides. There is no way in the world anyone can throw in a wet mattress.

The bobcat was fantastic in that sort of situation. Of course, I asked my friend for permission after I finished using it. You kick in and help. I don't know anyone who refused to help.

Everyone in the community who could pitch in did so in whatever way they could. All differences were put aside. You just got in and did it because there was a job to be done.

Floods have a different impact from the fires. Except for 2007, which took us all by surprise and came up very quickly overnight, generally, around here, you know the flood is coming, and you can prepare for it. There's not much you can do about it.

Whereas when the bigger fires are coming, you can prepare for it and do things. You can be busy and take your mind off any stress and worry.

I was pleased to see that efforts to build community resilience seem to be increasing. Again, this is not a criticism, but we're not very good at an agency level in building community resilience. I'd like to know if next time, we know how to be prepared for that. Things are getting better.

I don't know where that desire to help comes from. For example, the tavern is a place I go very occasionally, but I recognised that until the tavern and the village got cleaned up, we weren't ready for people to come back into the area. If the tavern, the shops, and the cafes take a big hit, that's going to impact all of us because if we lose those businesses, we're going to lose the town.

It's about helping people in the community. The people who owned the tavern at the time were my neighbours. I know them, they're good people. That's how Wollombi is.

The same thing happened in 2019. Those policy and operation decisions were made that the RFS wouldn't go to certain areas. The community just said we would go. They went to the places and saved houses.

It's good and bad. It worries me that people were putting themselves at risk, but that concern is being addressed now. I know the RFS is working towards working with private firefighting people. The RFS began with the community getting together.

In 2019, Braidwood was struggling for help from the RFS. They didn't have enough people, and they were literally burning them out. I went down and saw an area where this connection between the RFS and the private people, the farmers, and others worked really well. They talked to each other and told each other what they were doing and where they were.

But that's not universal across the state. That's what the RFS is trying to work towards. We're going back, reinventing the wheel, and coming full circle to where the RFS started, which amuses and delights me.

When the State Emergency Services (SES) came and said that everything must stop until we take control, they got a strong message back. 'Well, no, you're in the way. We're happy for you to help, but we're already doing it. Grab a broom, a shovel, pitch in.' To their credit, they didn't exert any authority once they got the message.

Cleaning up after a flood is a terrible, hard job.

There's undoubtedly sadness, especially for people who don't have insurance. You're trying to help them out as best you can and save whatever you can. But ultimately, it's just a big job.

It's good that you're working hard. You don't get time to have emotions. At the end, you think, thank God that's over, that's a job well done.

What always encouraged us is that community spirit. It was hard work, but we had a couple of laughs along the way. There's always a joke to be had along the way to keep people going. It builds those relationships.

As I said, some people have differences. They usually wouldn't talk to each other, but there they are, joking with each other. One fellow came up to me only about 18 months ago and said, 'You know, I'd always been told you're a bit of a bugger. You're actually a good guy.'

Gee, that made me pleased. He had a wrong impression of me. Then, seeing how I'd helped during the floods changed his opinion of me. My opinion of other people has probably changed, too. We know that people will chip in to help when the chips are down.

The floods are all different here. Each one behaves differently.

From all these events I've been involved in, I've learned that giving people the opportunity to talk is important. I think for many of them, it's the first time they've been given that permission to tell their story.

You let it all out, and some of the stories are amazing. It's heartbreaking. You can physically see and hear the emotion being let out, and that's great.

With the floods here, I don't know that that's happened much. There have been some meetings post-flood to discuss whether people have had the opportunity to vent their emotions or whether that was necessary.

I don't know of too many people who were dramatically affected to that point. I'm sure if things had gone badly and we'd had a loss of life or something like that, things would have been very different. Thankfully, that didn't happen. I know that in the distant past, there have been flood events where people have lost their lives, and that's had a very long-lasting impact.

People still occasionally talk about things that happened 30 years ago. They haven't forgotten that. Floods are strange things. They generally come up slowly and go down slowly, and there's not that adrenaline rush of panic with them that you get with other events.

Regarding the long-term impact of the 2022 floods, Wollombi is a funny place. There's a permanent population. Many people have weekenders here, and they generally come from Sydney.

The permanent population are probably used to it, it's just another flood. The weekender population don't have that knowledge and experience of floods reasonably regularly.

I think the effect on them would be varied. I'm sure some people thought they were not going through that again, so they sold up and left. Other people probably thought, well, that'll never happen again. We're okay. Let's pretend it never happened. The long-term impact is hard to say.

When I first came here, there were many small floods, and it was quite common for people who had to access the house to go across the creek. People would always prepare. Most of those people had a deep freeze with a lot of food stored in it because they knew they could be flooded in for three or four days until the water went down. They were self-sufficient, and no one had to worry about them too much.

That idea has been lost. We're now in a situation where people often run out of food after 12 hours and need assistance. It would be good if people moving into the area recognised the risk and got back into that habit. I would love it if they talked to their old-time neighbours about what's happened in the past. I'm pretty sure it doesn't always happen. Unfortunately, we're losing that experience. We're losing the real old-timers and their experience.

I've been to university and have a master's degree. I learned a lot through great mentors who taught me valuable things. Unfortunately, we lost a couple of them before I got a chance to absorb all their knowledge, which is incredibly disappointing.

That knowledge is important. As an example, and link to cultural burning, we've got a local here who, for a long time, was known as the local arsonist. Over time, I realised he knew what he was doing. He was burning in a way that was very similar to traditional cultural burning techniques.

I chatted with him, and I said, 'Who taught you how to burn?'

He said, 'Oh, my father.'

'Well, who taught him?'

'My grandfather.'

'Where did he learn? Wasn't he the first one here? Did you have many Aboriginal men working on the farm?'

'Oh yes, they worked for my grandfather.'

'Do you think they might have taught your grandfather how to burn?'

'Well, yes, they might have.'

It all comes together. Those techniques were passed down. But again, it's about those mentors. Things were done some time ago that seemed to impact mitigating flood outcomes.

The Wollombi Brook is a very interesting river system. I've got a book about it in the house. It was written by a couple of people from Newcastle Uni about 20- 25 years ago about the Wollombi Brook. One thing that stood out in that for me was a scientific explanation of how the flooding works. Don't quote me on this, but it was about the maximum flood level.

There is the one in 100-year flood level and the one in 500-year flood level. The one in 500-year flood level is about two or three times the one in 100-year flood level, except for two places in the world.

Those are the Wollombi Brook and a river in China, where it's about 12 times. It's a massive catchment that goes into very small river systems.

When we get floods, we really get floods. I laugh when people talk about replacing bridges around here. They say, 'Let's raise the bridge by a metre.' Well, the bridge is 20 metres underwater. That's not going to make any difference. There's not much to mitigate floods around here. We get them fast, and they're intense when we get them.

We need to learn the lessons of the past. I think the Catholic church in Wollombi is the second oldest Catholic church in Australia. It was originally built down on the banks of the creek. In about 1830-50, somewhere around there. After one big flood, they realised they'd made a mistake, and they pulled the whole thing apart and re-erected it further up on a hill.

There are many times we haven't learned that lesson. Don't build down in the floodplain. People are still doing it.

I was at the Wollombi Tavern in 2007. At that point, the water came up to the bar level, but we were able to wade in and carry a lot of valuable things out, like booze and cigarettes.

In 2022, it reached the ceiling level, and everything below that was inundated. It was a mess with mud everywhere. Using the high-pressure hose from the tanker, you could wash it out, and then ten minutes later, it dried off a bit, but it's still muddy. If you wash it out again, it's still muddy.

During the following renovations, much of the lining was removed from the wall. I suspect that they just couldn't get the mud out. It's a horrible job. Everything's wet, slimy, and smelly.

Cleanup is so much easier after a fire. With a flood, it's heartbreaking stuff. Having to throw things away when you've got pallet after pallet of beer or wine because it's technically spoiled, whether it is or not. It's such a waste.

It felt like we had the skip bins for months, and they were continually being filled up from around the district.

If I were to put together a checklist for people in flood-prone areas, I would say that if it's starting to rain, people living outside of the immediate flood zone, where we're not directly impacted, should stock up if they have the opportunity. Generally, people do that. Down in the village, places like that, where there's a good chance it's going under, people should start moving things.

It's more about awareness, and one of the big things that assisted us in 2022 was that prior to 2022, the Bureau of Meteorology installed river gauges so we could check the water levels. That made a huge difference because you could monitor from home and discuss with your neighbours where the water was rising and how fast it was rising.

At the top of the list would be keeping an eye on those gauges and understanding how they work.

There is little you can do before and during the flood. It's not possible. You can't stop the flood. You must just ride it out and make sure people are safe and aware.

Warnings are about the only thing you can do. The most important thing is post-flood recovery and assistance with the cleanup. For those areas where people are impacted mentally or physically, I think they need that opportunity to talk. It may well be that nobody needs to talk, but you need to give them that opportunity to vent whatever they're feeling.

I can understand why the agencies don't do it. Why would you put yourself up in front of a town meeting where you're going to be attacked? But you must do it. That's part of the job; you've got to wear that. If people are angry, let them be angry. Let them get it out.

This area bounced back well from floods. Get in, clean it up and move on. That's coming from an area that's used to floods.

However, I'm not sure you'd have the same thing in Broke and places like that, where people are not used to it.

It must come as an awful shock. You're just not prepared for it. 'That's never going to happen. Why should I even think about it?'

The best thing to offer people is encouragement to take matters into their own hands if they're not satisfied with the response and assistance they're getting. Go ahead and do it for yourself. They did that up in the Blue Mountains, and the results are spectacular. You don't get anything by sitting back and complaining. Take the bull by the horns.

It's all about taking a positive rather than a negative attitude following the event, rather than complaining about what's happened. What can we do? What can we learn from it? What can we do for the future?

BERNADETTE TOLSON

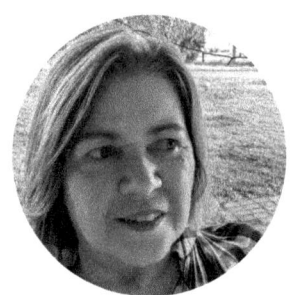

Bernadette lives with her husband, Max, on a property called Broke Estate on the outskirts of Broke. They have accommodation, a vineyard, and cattle on the property. They were on other side of the infamous road collapse that blocked of the local villages. Eventually they could get to Singleton but it was a few days before they could get into Broke.

'It was scary because we were very isolated. We were on an island because there was water all around us, and the road to Singleton was closed. Our neighbours were also blocked off from us. We thought if we did get stuck there, we could go up into the ceiling and onto the roof, but we didn't think the flood would get that high. We had to stay calm.'

Their house was not flooded but they had many other challenges on the property, including the need to rescue their livestock. Even so, they were able to observe what was happening around them.

'The connection to the village really came for us once the road opened, and we were able to go down and be part of the village and of that recovery check-in point at the community centre. It was like a war zone. It was very sad to see the devastation; it was dirty and wet. The sun was shining, and it was really eerie.'

The family's level of preparedness for natural disasters was tested and they realised the importance of better evacuation plans and resources.

BERNADETTE TOLSON

Bernadette believes Broke village is bouncing back but also bouncing forward, and describes the significance of wellness initiatives, community involvement, and support services in fostering connectedness and resilience.

I grew up in Broke and left when I was 18 to go to the big city of Sydney. Then, I moved to Victoria and returned to Hunter Valley in 2012. Little did I know that we would buy a property at the end of the street where I grew up, but apparently that happens quite often. We purchased the property, Broke Estate, in 2012, and we have an acreage where we run cattle, have a vineyard, and accommodation. It's a beautiful property.

Broke itself is a beautiful place for us. We love our farm and have spent much time and energy restoring it. It was a very rundown property. My husband works on the farm. He works away, but he's the main person. I'm the assistant manager when he's away. We have two wonderful children who live in Adelaide but are very involved in the property. It's our special place.

My flood story begins on the Sunday, before the floods. Max and I were down in the vineyard, and we looked across to the Telstra towers over near Margan Wine but we couldn't see them because of the rain. We thought, oh, there's another big rainstorm coming.

I went to work on Monday morning, and when I got to the intersection of Broke and Cessnock Road, I looked down towards Wollombi, and the water was over the road. I had seen this before and wasn't too perturbed about it. After a long meeting that finished at 1 pm, I thought I should check the BOM to see what was happening with the weather.

Of course, all the hazard alerts said that the roads were closed and flooded. I left work at about 1:20 pm and went home but couldn't get past Hermitage Road. On the way, I observed the flooding in Nulkaba, and the Christian school, St. Philips, was entirely flooded around it like an island.

Luckily, it was school holidays, so children were not affected. I had to go home via Singleton but didn't get home until after 3 pm, so it was a very long, wet journey. When I got home, we had water coming up onto the property.

It was a bit surreal and unexpected; there weren't any warnings. Max and I went down to the fire station, where we met a wonderful person, Robbie, who said, 'If you've got cattle, you should go home and get them up because the water's coming fast, and it's going to be a big flood.'

Before we went to the fire station, I thought there must have been a broken water main on the main road because cars were going past and splashing everywhere. But it wasn't a water main; the river was already coming, and the water was over the road by the time we got home.

Our property was where the Broke Road collapsed, segregating one side of the town from the other. Initially, water was across the road separating Broke and Singleton, but gradually, the water dried up on the Singleton side. We could go to Singleton, but we could not get into the village itself.

The main thing we thought about was our cattle. We had a cow in calf that we needed to rescue and 12 young heifers down in the water that we had to rescue.

Max set out on his four-wheel motorbike, which got flooded and damaged, and we had to replace it. It was a miracle the cow and the calf followed him out of the stockyards. Then he returned home for some wire cutters and went back to cut the fence and get the heifers out.

We were happy that we had rescued them. It wasn't about the value of the cattle; it was about the lives of our livestock. We would have hated to see those cattle float away. We'd been there for the birth of every one of those calves, and they were precious to us.

We managed to get the 12 heifers near the house, then they were safe. By this stage it was getting dark, then the water just progressed up to the house itself and stopped—thankfully. That was about 1 am. In the meantime, we had many phone calls from friends interstate telling us that the floods were bad. We didn't know how bad they were because we didn't have any communication.

The power had gone out, and it was dark, so we couldn't watch the news. We were very mindful not to use our telephones to save the batteries. Luckily, we remembered we had some battery packs in the shed and could charge our telephones. It was a wait-and-see game, and I wondered what was happening everywhere else.

It was scary because we were very isolated. We were on an island because there was water all around us, and the road to Singleton was closed. Our neighbours were also blocked off from us. We thought if we did get stuck there, we could go up into the ceiling and onto the roof, but we didn't think the flood would get that high. We had to stay calm.

We'd learned a lot of resilience from the bushfires and needed a safety plan. My daughter in Adelaide was amazing; she was on the phone constantly, making us think about our evacuation future and what we should do. We've got two beautiful dogs. How are we going to manage the dogs? They were going to go with us, no doubt.

Max had previously had surgery, so he was still recuperating and shouldn't have been wandering around in dirty water. We had to relax amid the stress.

How did we manage that? Apart from cold cups of tea, it was the phone calls from friends. My sister was a great person. Throughout the night, she kept calling and checking in on us. It was around having that connection with someone who understood—not the floods, but understood us as human beings. That was how we managed stress; she talked us through the disaster.

I had great delight in going out every hour and marking the water as it was coming up to the house. My mother used to do that many years ago. That was, for me, a task to keep my mind at ease. I sent Max to bed at about 1 am because I thought he needed some rest. I went and cleared the shed out because I had a lot of memorabilia in the shed that I was worried might flood, so I was out there busy lifting it up onto tables.

It was about daylight when you could see that the water on the bricks was not going any higher and was stable.

I think we've done better at preparation since the flood. Most people in any flooded area, and particularly in Broke, would probably have better evacuation plans, even though this was an incredibly fast flood. Be more prepared. We thought we were prepared, things like acquiring a generator—we still need to get it—so we have power. We certainly had plenty of food.

When I first came to the country to live, my friend said, 'You must always have lots of food in your freezer,' which we do. We lived on frozen vegetables and frozen fish for a week. But be prepared emotionally and have evacuation plans. Since the disaster, most people in Broke now know who the significant people would be to call in an emergency. Whereas before, it was a little bit vague. That's a positive thing that's come out of the floods. We're more connected.

Some days later, on Wednesday, we received several phone calls from the SES and the fire brigade about evacuation. We requested and were approved to stay because we had water and food, and we were concerned that, as the fences had been washed away, once the water went down, the cattle could escape.

We didn't bother anyone in the community because we were safe, and the only thing we wanted was water. We didn't have any fresh drinking water, which was delivered to us as soon as possible. I did collect rainwater. I had all my basins outside in the yard collecting water.

The connection to the village really came for us once the road opened, and we were able to go down and be part of the village and of that recovery check-in point at the community centre. It was like a war zone. It was very sad to see the devastation; it was dirty and wet. The sun was shining, and it was really eerie.

It was just incredible. The first shock was people's personal belongings on the streets, but then the place was buzzing. People had many mixed emotions, but there was food, and there were people, such as the police and the politicians. You name it, they were there to help out. We just felt very welcomed driving into town on our four-wheel motorbike without any helmets and with hi-vis jackets on. Driving down the road on a quad bike and not seeing a car was weird.

I didn't know a lot of residents because the village had changed a lot— there were only a couple of people I really knew. But I got to know some amazing people in that community. Then I realised what a very well-connected village it was. The people there were working very closely together. As I said, there were some mixed emotions. There were chaplains from the army walking around the street, wanting to support people who needed it. There was a lot of support there and fellowship.

Broke people offered support to each other, but some fantastic services came in after a few days and supported the village and the people. People came from Lismore with learned experience. The Salvation Army, the Red Cross, and Land Services were there. Plus Centrelink and Resilience New South Wales. Initially, they were in the hall, the community centre, but when that became a virtual shopping centre and a work area for jobs to be done, the services ended up in the local Catholic church.

I remember going there one day just because everyone else was there and stood at the door. We didn't need anything, but the Salvation Army lady said, 'Come and sit down,' we had a chat, and she gave us a voucher for Bunnings, which was amazing. We didn't expect that. But many people were in need, and they knew what to do. They were incredible people.

What was most disturbing for me was the break in the road, not just for us in the village but for people who used that road every day. There are literally thousands who used that over a week, and they couldn't commute to work. It was a long journey around to go to work for the people in Broke itself. Luckily, it was school holidays, so the children didn't need to go to school, but for them to go to work in Singleton or go into Singleton to their GP or bank or any services, they had to go around the long way. That was stressful for people. It was stressful in their cars, time away from their home, where they wanted to be.

Because we were isolated physically, it was frustrating that we couldn't get in there earlier and help. By the time we were able to get to the village, things had been so well organised. I could stop and chat with people, as a resident, if they wanted to chat. But it was the presence of turning up for the wonderful community meals at night, having friendships with those people and acknowledging that we were safe. We didn't have house damage, but we could come and support people sitting around a meal. Food is always a wonderful healer.

After the flood, because ours is a working property, we're still working on the recovery, but we had fantastic help from Beyond Ballooning. They regularly land their balloons on our property in autumn and winter. That's looking at not just the people in Broke but also the services; the tourism industry beyond Broke was damaged because they couldn't come and bring their balloon flights. Beyond Ballooning purchased some sort of grader or digger to help make a driveway for us. Four or five guys came initially to do some fencing and repair some fences, and then they brought their digger to make a driveway for us.

Then we had the army. There were five amazing young guys, all about 20 years old, who had just finished the first part of their military training. I really enjoyed working on the property with them. We had a wonderful day. They talked about their girlfriends, the army, and where they went to school. The sun was shining, and they were covered in mud.

They did a great job, they were fantastic. Down the track, we had Blaze Aid come and help with the fencing. They were incredible. Then, lots of friends came to help restore the fences and the grapes, getting the grapes to stand up again because they had been knocked over.

Once the property dried out, the vines started to shoot because it was springtime. The flood vintage was a bit of a disaster. Production was low, but the next year, we picked up again. But they were very resilient vines, they bounced back.

It's been a slow process for most people to put their properties back together. Some were able to move back into their homes quite quickly. Others are still waiting for their homes to be rebuilt. There are different levels of people being able to move back and recover, and that's probably difficult for some who are still not back in their homes. For the properties, it took a long time for fences to be restored, livestock to be returned, and grass to grow again for the livestock.

The village has coped very well as time has gone on. They're quite a resilient group of people. Tourism is back. We're looking forward to our Bicentenary at the end of the year in October. That's bringing a lot of the community together. We've just been nominated as finalists in the Top Tourism Town award, and people are taking a lot of pride in their homes and front yards.

There is a buzz. There are a lot of significant people in the village. Maybe it's the guy on the digger who has done a lot of work and is very social; it's networking. The fire brigade people and the Broke Residents Group are fantastic.

It's bounced back, and it's bouncing forward. There appears to be a lot more connectedness in the village. That goes back to the early days after the initial emergency centre was disbanded when there was a big community dinner for everyone. It was a fantastic show of people who all turned up.

That was the beginning of the change of moving forward. Since then, there's been ongoing funding for wellness sessions, yoga, mindfulness sessions, and morning teas. There's more connectedness in those group settings than before, and more people are aware of them.

What I learned through this experience is that we are a lucky community. There were no major injuries or fatalities. It was a natural disaster, and floods happen. Unfortunately for us, it was possibly the biggest one ever. But we're fortunate to be a lucky community in a lucky country with services and support in place. It's important for everyone to use those and not to feel isolated. For people who were feeling isolated and did not want to go to the community centre, there was someone to take them aside and encourage them to go and visit and be part of things. There was the understanding of different people's emotional needs and mental health needs that may have been pre-existing and then raised their nasty heads when these disasters happen.

Hopefully, it never happens again, but if it does, the community is already doing things. I am part of a couple of committees in Broke, working on different things. The Residents Committee is looking at having contact with people in certain areas, which would be helpful.

Like I said, I didn't make phone calls because I was aware that a lot of people were worse off than me. However, in the future, there will be one contact in a designated area, about five throughout the area. That person would take phone calls, screen, help people, and keep them up to date with what was happening. I would like to take on one of those roles.

Personally, I'm probably not as anxious now about floods because certainly when the next flood, the next heavy rain, came, I was very anxious. Overall, I'm more empathetic around other people and how they respond to disasters.

I think Broke will continue to grow and be a beautiful village, but still with a very rural aspect. We've got this little tight-knit community, but around it, we've got some outstanding properties, which, as you're driving, are in a beautiful setting.

On my property, we still have a lot of devastation. I haven't mentioned that we had a massive wash away of the riverbank. We hope that someday it will be restored. We're not sure how that will happen without hundreds of thousands of dollars spent. Our property will continue to be our little treasure. Fortunately, we had a glamping site on our riverbank that survived. It had been put back on hold in March because of the floods. We were ready to have our first opening and guests a couple of weeks after the floods.

It had been a long project that my son had been working on, and amazingly, it was the only thing standing on the property. If you see aerial photos, it is one little white tent. We want to have more glamping sites, not on the river but up on higher ground, and continue with our accommodation opportunities. Personally, I'd like to have some time off work and potter around the property.

In conclusion, I'd like to acknowledge the support the politicians, Dave Layzell and Dan Repacholi provided to the community. They were there for every meeting after the event. But before their appearance, you know, people like Evelyn Hardy set up the emergency centre. Mick McCardle stepped up to the role of heading up the operations. Then, I met a guy in the hall at the community centre. He came from nowhere and said he'd like to help. He ended up managing all the whiteboards.

I couldn't believe it. There were five whiteboards, and everyone had a number with a name next to it. Those guys and the mining company came on board, and they were designating job numbers to people. That was incredible. I couldn't believe that could happen. None of them had ever had that experience before. There was a lady, Angela, who lived across the river, and she had to be evacuated. Her place was flooded.

She set up a GIVIT Foundation fundraising group. The money was then allocated to people who needed it through a committee. She was also excellent at social media.

All those people like Kathleen and her team at the fire brigade who worked endlessly day and night. All those volunteers.

BERNADETTE TOLSON

DR ROB GORDON

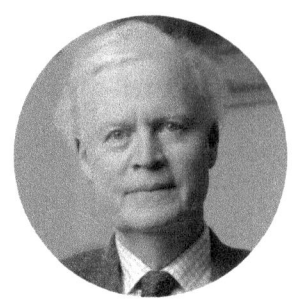

Dr Rob Gordon is an experienced psychologist who specialises in disaster trauma. He explains the effects on the human psyche of trauma from disasters and describes strategies for recovery. Rob is warm and compassionate, and his examples, which all come from his experience over many years, illustrate the complexity of the human response to tragic events and explain why it can take many years to recover.

For Rob, having strong support and social networks is the most crucial ingredient of learning to heal from this type of trauma.

'In these close-knit communities, people transmit information to each other. It becomes a process of collective learning.'

My story began when I was part of a Royal Children's Hospital team working on the Ash Wednesday fires in the Macedon area. I realised that nobody knew what we should be trying to do with people involved in disasters of this sort.

I gradually became aware that a whole range of other problems happen to people. One of the biggest comes from a disaster being an unprecedented event. Most people have not been through one. If they have, they probably never fully comprehended it. So that doesn't help them with the next one unless it was a minor scare that gives them experience.

I learned that it was essential to listen to people and find out what was going on for them without making assumptions. Over the years, I've gradually seen patterns emerging. I want to emphasise that because a disaster is a social event by definition, everyone in that community is somehow affected. That creates a social dimension to the problem that we don't usually see in routine mental health situations with stress and so forth.

When a tragedy such as a fatal road accident or a criminal event occurs, and they occur all the time, a specific number of people are affected, but not so much the people around them. They are then available to become supporters. In a disaster, there's a whole range of problems.

I remember working with people after the Canberra fires, and a woman told me that nearly all the houses in her street burnt except hers. She had lived there for years in a warm, supportive, close-knit community. Now she had empty blocks around her, which would take years to rebuild.

No one expects that, so it becomes part of the problem. People have a range of expectations. They might have built a house before, and their timeframe for building is measured around when they choose to do it. They've got the money and been through all the preliminaries. But if everyone in the community is trying to rebuild a house, it's completely different.

There's a very tangible experience in the initial stage, including three elements that I think are most important. The first is trauma, the word we use for a psychological injury that comes from having an experience that exceeds your previous experience and assumptions. These experiences are often associated with intense feelings of helplessness and involve a serious threat to yourself or others.

I've learned that what is traumatic is not necessarily what happens if bad things happen, but the trauma injury is created by what you think is going to happen because that determines your reaction. In any natural disaster environment, there will be many people who go through experiences where they think they might be killed, their loved ones might have died, or other terrible things have happened. That stimulates a deep-seated reorganisation of yourself to try and accept it, take it on and deal with it, but without understanding what you've done.

Those adjustments often remain in place until the person realises what they did. A simple example I remember is a woman telling me that on Ash Wednesday when people were on the reserve in Mount Macedon. They wouldn't do this now, but a blackened, traumatised fire crew staggered in off their truck and went around to people, saying, 'Your house is all right. Yours is gone. Yours is gone. Yours is okay. We dunno about yours.'

The woman who told me this said people spent the rest of the night grieving their house. But when things settled down, maybe the next day or so, they went out slowly and carefully in their car, and as they came around the corner, their house was untouched. She said, 'I'm ashamed to say it, but I felt a pang of disappointment.' That disappointment is significant.

There are stories from the Second World War when people got a message about their loved ones. In those days, it was probably a telegram saying that your husband was missing in action, presumed dead. Then three years later, he rocks up and knocks on the door, 'I'm alive, I'm here.' Those marriages often didn't last; the kids didn't recognise the fathers, and so on.

So, this profound reorganisation goes on at an unconscious level where we're generally not operating. And that trauma is a critical issue, and it's varied because we can have all sorts of different traumas.

The second problem is loss. And loss causes grief, but there can be different kinds of losses.

These were all my learning experiences. A few years into the recovery in Mount Macedon, a woman said there used to be a beautiful place on Mount Macedon with a lovely view and surrounded by natural beauty. A little creek ran through it. 'Whenever I was sad, I would go and sit there, and I'd look over the mountain for a couple of hours, and I'd feel better. But that's all burnt now. It's all gone.' So, she's really lost her mental health resource. And she really felt that, but it's very hard to talk about.

This woman did not lose her house. But loss comes in, whatever the loss. It could be the loss of friends. Think of the woman in Canberra. Loss of community, environment, property, loss of many things that ultimately mean something and therefore are part of you. Then one of the significant challenges is, 'How do I still feel myself when I've lost everything that's part of my history?'

The broad spectrum of losses means it's hard for people to understand each other. Another story that comes to mind is talking to a flooded community in Central Victoria; I remember the scene vividly. It was in a racing clubroom with rows of chairs, and I was talking about what people might go through and how they could look after themselves.

A couple of rows back, I noticed a woman sitting there with a very sad face, and after a time, she put up her hand and said, 'Excuse me, is it possible that people who weren't affected could also feel upset?'

I said, 'Yes, of course. I spoke about some of these things.'

She said, 'Thank you. Well, we were affected; our shed was flooded.'

A woman was sitting behind her who also looked pretty upset. I mentioned that she had lost everything, and this other woman said my shed was flooded. The woman behind her literally rolled her eyes as if to say, 'Oh, you poor thing - your shed is flooded; I'm so sorry for you.'

I was looking at her sadness and thought, what can I say? And I just said, 'What do you keep in your shed?

She said, 'All the effects from my mother's estate. She died a month or so before the flood.'

How could anyone understand her sadness and that she's entitled to recovery support unless they talk? But soon as she spoke up, everyone would say, 'Oh gee, that's pretty tough.'

There is a social effect that I first read about in a book published in the 1960s in America by a very famous sociologist in America called Robert Merton, and he was probably one of the first people to start looking at disasters.

He noticed that there was a tendency for people to benchmark their impact against the most severe tragic impact in the community. If they didn't have anything like that, they didn't feel entitled to ask for help. 'Don't worry about me. Go see poor Rob; he's lost everything.' Or 'Don't worry about Evelyn; she's only lost this, that and the other. Rob's got the problem.'

Merton called that relative deprivation. What's behind that is that we constantly make sense of our experiences in everyday life by drawing comparisons with the people around us. After all, the whole notion of normality is based on that comparison. If everybody I know thinks this, I'm not crazy—I'm just normal.

There's a process whereby when everyone's gone through this huge experience, they contract into a tight, what I call a state of fusion. Tight, strong, supportive and rushing around helping each other in the early days. But as time passes, these differences emerge when people often lock into their perspective.

One of the problems of the recovery period is that there's often a period of social turmoil and conflict, sometimes with very bitter and destructive comments. With social media, we know you can say whatever you like, and everybody will know. Then some very emotional thoughtless things are said, which are extremely wounding.

I have a story about a man I met five or six years ago after a flood. He told me he was in Ash Wednesday with his young family. They're all grown up now, but he had grown up with my cousin, who was about the same age. They were best friends. Their families went on holiday together. They got girlfriends, went out together and got married at the same time. They shared their lives completely together and then lived in different communities.

But his house burnt down, and everything was in turmoil with him. A few days later, his cousin rang up and said, 'Oh, you weren't affected by that terrible fire, were you?'

He said, 'yeah, we lost everything.'

His cousin said, 'Oh my goodness. I'm so sorry to hear it. You are alright, though, aren't you?'

He said it would be alright. Then from that day to this, he's never heard from him again. It's a very dramatic story, but many people feel frightened of emotion, suffering and trauma, and they shy away from it.

Now, I immediately thought of the research done since the 1950s on mental health, which showed that good social support is the number one protective factor for mental and physical health. So, just when you want to maximise the stability of your familiar support system, it falls away.

There's been outstanding research from the United States showing the number one predictor of both the speed and adequacy of recovery. It is not the amount of money spent, the amount of infrastructure built or the political connections. It's what they call social capital, which is the relationships you have with people.

There are various sorts of relationships that you need. Studies in Japan after the Fukushima earthquake showed these relationships don't just predict the recovery in all the different communities—they also predicted the death rate. Because where communities had high social capital and good relationships, they didn't wait for the authorities to warn them that the tsunami was coming. Anyone who saw them contacted everybody, and they had arrangements where people jumped over the fence, picked up the old fella next door, put him on their shoulders, and went up the nearest hill.

This leads me to a significant experience: when a disaster occurs, it always involves physical events. It's a little bit different when you see one of those bus crashes, which I've worked on a number of. You know, those sorts of things where there's often very high traumatic experience, deaths, injuries, but the physical damage is not significant. Then you've got a focus on the psychological experience.

But when the physical situation is totally demolished, the focus is on the physical situation. Even if people have died, if you've lost loved ones, but your house has gone, you've got to get going on your new home as soon as you can.

Therefore, there is a tendency for everybody—including the cabinet ministers—to focus on the physical, until they've been educated. When you have people like politicians and decision-makers who've had some experience, that's very helpful. They've learned things, but the initial instinct is that everybody thinks this is all about rebuilding.

Yet people have had life-changing experiences which are like a rupture to the flow of their life, which brings in the third factor, which took me ten years or so to start to understand. We had trauma, then loss leading to grief.

What you lose is not just an object that's part of you, part of your identity, but the third one is that people's lives are disrupted through trauma.

When you lose your physical infrastructure, suddenly, you have a massive new task. I often use this example with people doing training. Imagine you go home tonight and find a huge tree has fallen on your bathroom and completely demolished it.

Have you got time to go through the insurance, builders, planning, and local government, then choose the tiles and so on and so forth? Or are your lives already full? They're already full. Okay. But you're going to have to do that, aren't you? Or you won't be able to have a shower. So, what are you going to put aside? You can't stop going to work, you won't have the money to pay for the bathroom.

So, you put aside everything that's dispensable. Talking to your wife, for instance, playing with your kids, visiting your in-laws, going for a run, talking to your friends. You haven't got time for any of that stuff for a few months.

Then what happens is that people's lives become reorganised around the priority of getting the job done. That's what healthy, competent, capable people do. They focus on what must be done, but they can't do it fast enough because their assumptions about how long it will take are based on if a tree fell on their bathroom, but of course, it's different. And so, their assumptions don't fit what's going to unfold.

We've done research in Victoria, which shows that anything that creates high emotion in people post-disaster means their brains go into that survival-oriented stress zone. They become incapable of using their higher mental faculties, prioritising strategic planning, long-term judgements and problem-solving. They go into, 'I've got to get this done now' mode, which often means they get angry and upset, get into conflict and don't achieve things.

Then, when they're very stressed, they often can't even get on with their processes, so their recovery stalls. And people will often say, 'I haven't been able to do anything this month.'

For example, I talk about how you can't make decisions in this state of stress. You can't even remember things. I know I've hit the mark when I say you'll realise when you're stressed because you go to the bedroom to get something, but you can't remember what it is by the time you get there.

Then you go back to your study and realise you can't read your computer screen. And you go back to look for your glasses and can't find them anywhere. You spend half an hour looking, and then as you walk back down the corridor, you pass a mirror that shows they're sitting on your head. We all get into this kind of disorganisation, and people drive themselves mad.

The real problem is that their recovery stalls. What would they need to get out of that? Go to a barbecue with the community and eat half-cooked sausages and laugh together. Tell jokes. Maybe have someone come along and play music or a comedian, as laughing together brings them out of the stress, and their brains restart.

I was talking about this in a town significantly affected by Black Saturday, and I went back there about six months later and did a follow-up. The bloke who ran the local caravan park approached me and said, 'I heard you last time, and I realised you were talking about me; I couldn't get anything done. I talked to my wife, and we took the family to Bali for two or three weeks. When I returned, I achieved more in three days than in three weeks.'

People don't realise that when we disrupt our lives, we lose all the patterns we've achieved to make our life manageable, keep ourselves on the ball, balance recreation, and so on. What's really lost are our routines. Once we lose routines, we go into a state of improvising daily life. You don't have to think about what you're doing when you're in a routine. You can be processing all sorts of things. You can get up, have breakfast, get dressed, and drive to work for half an hour. Many people said they missed that commute because it was their time of mulling and processing.

If we don't do that, we can't get things into perspective. We can't pull in various bits and hold them all together. But we do that without thinking about everyday life. We don't realise we've lost it because we are so focused, and stress produces this tunnel vision on our problems. All the resources we need are falling away.

When I started analysing routines, I realised we form routines around what's important to us. The example I give is a couple who want to be good parents. They fall into a habit that when the kids go off and do their homework after dinner and the parents tidy up the kitchen, they talk about how they will manage the weekend and deal with school problems.

Maybe they have a cup of tea together for a few minutes or half an hour and coordinate their parenting. Then they put the kids to bed, pay the bills, and go to bed. They formed a pattern where they would do that a few times a week, either after dinner or on Saturday afternoons when the kids played sports.

That's a routine where they coordinate their parenting. Now all you need for them to lose that completely is to plonk the family in a caravan for eighteen months. They haven't got space or a routine. They're squabbling over everything all the time.

Then you get a ten-year-old girl who tells her parents to stop arguing because she's got a test tomorrow. 'Dad, you sit down there, Mum, you sit down there and just be quiet. I've got homework to do.' The parents do it because they want their kids to have the homework. This ten-year-old girl is running the family, isn't she? The parents lose self-awareness of their stress state, and so when they move into their new house, she's now twelve or thirteen and not doing what she's told. That's because she's been running the family with these immature parents who have lost the plot. The loss of routines means we lose the values that the routines have been framed around and were embodied in their way of life. This is a significant area of loss that often occurs in the second and third years when people's lives are getting very tatty.

This brings us to the simple idea that the losses that occur in a disaster are, broadly speaking, reversible. Eventually, they'll have a house again.

Most people won't end up living under a bridge. It may never be as good a house, and their lives might never have the same structure as before, but they will live somewhere and have that frame of life.

I call that a reversible loss. They won't have their heirlooms, and the lady who lost her mother's stuff will never get that back. But as one woman told me, when she looked back seven years later, they realised they hadn't paid attention to the family relationships. She said she and her husband are still together but are just good friends. They've lost the intimacy of their marriage, and they don't know where it went because they were so busy all the time, so they drifted apart. Her fourteen-year-old daughter, at the time, is okay and is now at university, but they don't see her much because she's gone into her friendship network.

She said, 'The one I feel sorry for is my seven-year-old son at the time, who's now fourteen. He was a happy, outgoing boy with friends at school, enjoying learning. Now he's a lonely isolate with no friends at the school.'

I've had other couples who separated because it just didn't seem to work.

Research in the United States has shown us that the essence of resilience and what enables us to adjust to trauma are two things. Firstly, to be clear about the values important in our life and the qualitative features of our life, and secondly, to preserve social networks. None of us will do it alone without costing something very dear to us. For some people, it'll be physical health. For some people, it'll be mental health. For others, it'll be the loss of direction in their lives.

What's going to hold it all together is to preserve the quality of life, the structure of your life, and the values it pinned on, and to maintain that together with your community.

I've noticed that in a natural disaster, the research shows us that somewhere between about five and twenty per cent of people with severe trauma might need professional help, but everyone else has a bad experience. Most of them will muddle through if they've got a good social network and can talk together over a few years.

Any fissures, cleavages and ruptures in the community damage the structure they need to allow this communication of experience. With the communication of experience comes this sort of, 'Oh, I didn't realise that was happening for you. Oh, you poor thing.' Everyone moves out of their egocentric state in stress because stress is a mechanism for their problems.

You'll see the whole community will move together through this. Maybe it'd be good to get a talk from somebody who can give them some understanding of these things occasionally, but they don't all need a clinical session. When we come to the idea of resilience, those people who seem to do it better are those who have an instinctive sense that, 'I've lost everything. I will have a long, difficult time, but I've got to hang onto what's important. I've got to hang onto my relationships. I've got to hang onto the quality of life. I must ensure my kids continue to see their friends and have good experiences. We've got to hold onto recreational pursuits and the things that gave our lives meaning.'

To draw that together, I think what you see is a sort of natural process that goes like this:

When the impact occurs, people go into an initial survival state and rush around trying to survive. Then if they're not careful, they keep rushing for about six months and have utterly exhausted themselves. That will stop when they've got stable temporary arrangements.

They've got somewhere to live, figured out their insurance problems, and are making plans.

Next, they go into this long, gruelling, enduring, stressful situation of the entire recovery process, which will take years. They don't think so, but it will gradually take years. There's this emotional turmoil when people are exhausted, and this is when people's lives are at risk.

The one thing I would emphasise is staying involved in your community, even if you don't usually go along to community events. Encourage the community leaders—they're often affected too—and any agencies that come in to help run social events, entertainments opportunities to talk about their problems, engage in collective bargaining with governments, etc.

Work together and have a comfortable environment where people can hang around and talk around some food. Come early. This is where neighbourhood and community centres are crucial, but not everyone goes. Everyone that does go will do better. Then, when they have finally rebuilt, people take stock because you can't stop and think until you've moved into your new house.

Some people have a problem attaching to the new house. Their friends say from outside the area, 'Oh, aren't you lucky with the new house? I wish I had a new house.'

But people say, 'I didn't want this new house. I don't like living here. It feels like a motel. I loved my old house.' Then they don't invite them again, so what happens is that the meaning of the experience starts to come to the fore when they're no longer rushing around trying to fix everything up.

I call this the identity crisis period. Who am I? Are my life plans still relevant? Are the goals I had for my life still relevant, or am I changed? People do sometimes change. Often, we talk about how post-traumatic growth shifts towards more intangible, qualitative values in life, such as valuing relationships. If people can do this identity crisis stuff and work out, okay, so they've got a slightly different plan, 'I'm now clear that I'm not going to work three jobs and try and get a very expensive car and a speed boat. I'm just going to spend that time valuing my family 'cause we're all still alive, and that's wonderful.'

Once they've got that and they settle in, after another couple of years, they often go through a period of profound emotional exhaustion. 'I don't feel like going anywhere, don't feel like doing anything.'

I say, 'Well, that's unsurprising because you've been working hard in that survival mode. Then you've worked very hard for several years. In rebuilding and getting everything going, you've been working hard psychologically to work out all this new stuff. You deserve a rest.'

I call that stage recovery from recovery. It's essential to follow those cues. Tell your friends you are going to hibernate for a little while. 'I love you all, I'll be back, but I just need time to myself.'

I remember one woman who was very well connected in her country community, who got to the point where she would hide in her wardrobe because her friends would come around to visit. They were worried about her. In the mornings, after all the family had gone off to work and school, they'd see a car in the garage. They'd knock, and she wouldn't be there. Then they'd knock on the windows and doors, asking where she was.

She said, 'All I could do was shut myself in the wardrobe until they left.' It's better to understand that this is a stage and tell people.

It's better to start breaking up these phases. Start resting and processing in the first phase and do the long grind a bit slower. Take more time, go to Queensland now and again or enjoy yourself and value being with your family. Then go to community events and talk about life.

You'll be doing the identity work, so all these stages merge. This way, you don't allow it to be side-tracked by all the external things that say it's all about the physical infrastructure. When you do that, people come out at the end, saying, 'I'm a very different person than I was before. I never wanted to go through it.'

This is where I like the Kintsugi idea, you've got beautiful golden metallic fillings in the cracks. Once it's repaired it's very strong again, and I think the more people understand the journey, the better they can do it when it does arise.

Timing is crucial. It's very hard to get people's attention when they're in the first phase. They're too busy to come to meetings. But I've also had the experience of going to various communities, and I would go quite often, maybe every few months, to places.

In the fourth year after Black Saturday, I went to one community I had previously visited several times. Before the meeting, a woman approached me and said, 'I'm so pleased to finally get to one of your meetings.'

This is four years later. 'I've never managed to get there before because there are always too many other things, but many things people have told me have been enormously helpful. Thank you very much.'

Realise that in these close-knit communities, people transmit information to each other. It becomes a process of collective learning. When that happens, you get filtering out of information so that people draw on a collective understanding.

That can come from someone like me who's spent many years following it through, but it also comes from people telling their stories from other disasters. You know, often the most helpful thing is that people from the last disaster come along to the next one. When they're out the other side and come and share their experience and say do this, and don't do this, and so on. Some organisations provide group education sessions, but that's the main thing.

Of course, there's also reading stories or looking at videos. I know that there are about sixty videos of me telling this stuff on YouTube. I think I've repeated the same thing over again for decades, but everyone tells me that it's different because I'm probably learning things all the time.

When you talk to other people who've been through it, ask them questions, and get them to attend a community meeting. The most effective learning will happen through personal contact. Once you give words to something that connects to a person's experience, they say, 'Ah, yes, that's it, I understand it.' Then they can make good decisions and look after themselves.

I think a factor of resilience plays into trauma, and it has to do with our assumptions about life. Assumptions are formed by the repeated experiences of things being the same. I often illustrate that when I'm talking to groups and say, 'Did any of you consider whether this building you're in is built to earthquake standards, if we have an earthquake in fifteen minutes?' They never have unless they come from Christchurch because they don't happen here. If we haven't experienced this, it's not part of our assumptions.

Trauma is an experience that violates our assumptions about ourselves, nature, the world, other people, the seasons, anything. And it's like they get ripped, they get torn, and they have to be rebuilt. Now, post-traumatic stress is to rebuild the assumptions around the fact that this will happen, so I can never relax. I never feel safe. I always wait for it to happen again.

But the proper healing is to rebuild the assumption that says these things can happen.

It may never happen to me again, but it can happen. That means I need to live with that background, understand that there can be emergencies of all sorts, and have some knowledge about what I should do to keep myself and my loved ones safe. In that way, we can normalise emergencies.

I read some diaries about the Blitz in London as part of my research. There was a project there asking people throughout the community to keep diaries. If you read those diaries, they would be full of bombing raids. 'Oh, it was terrible bombing last night. Mrs Blog, around the corner, died, and these houses were broken. How can these Germans do this to us?'

But after a while, it was normalised, and the diary entry says, 'It was a terrible night last night. But I've been talking to Mrs Smith around the corner, who has a wonderful recipe for making birthday cakes from sump oil and beeswax. And I'm going to try it for my little boy's birthday.' That sort of thing.

I'm making a joke, but they're all about innovating the domestic routines around rationing and privation. These women were holding their families together. And that was the task they were working on. And the Blitz just became the background situation.

Of course, it would be the focus if their house was destroyed, or they lost people. But we all have this capacity, and I think we are in a stage where we must reset our assumptions around climate. Reset them; I think of it as in a state of poise. For instance, when you are poised standing on a train. I used to travel to the hospital by train for years, and I found that if I stood with my feet slightly apart and my knees slightly flexed in the train when I didn't get a seat, I could stand there in a poised way and read a book because otherwise, it's very boring.

To be poised is to be ready to respond. I think we can live our lives with poise in that way, but we've got to keep our eyes on the ball. I think the community is currently struggling with that. Many people don't want to let go of their assumptions or disagree with climate change, while others are jumping ahead, so this is a process of transition as a community. Mother Earth will have to find a new normal, which'll be disruptive. We need to be willing to go with it.

For more information, search Rob Gordon, Disaster Psychologist, on YouTube for many videos others have put up.

Contact: rob@robgordon.com.au

www.ingramcontent.com/pod-product-compliance
Lightning Source LLC
Chambersburg PA
CBHW062048290426
44109CB00027B/2767